# ＳENSUAL ＭASSAGE

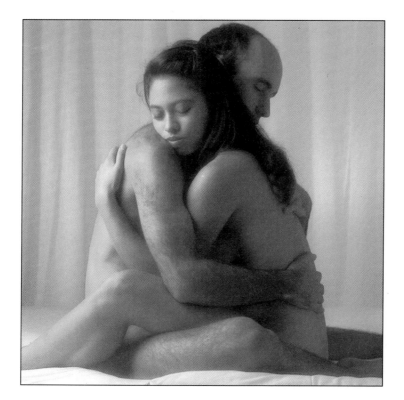

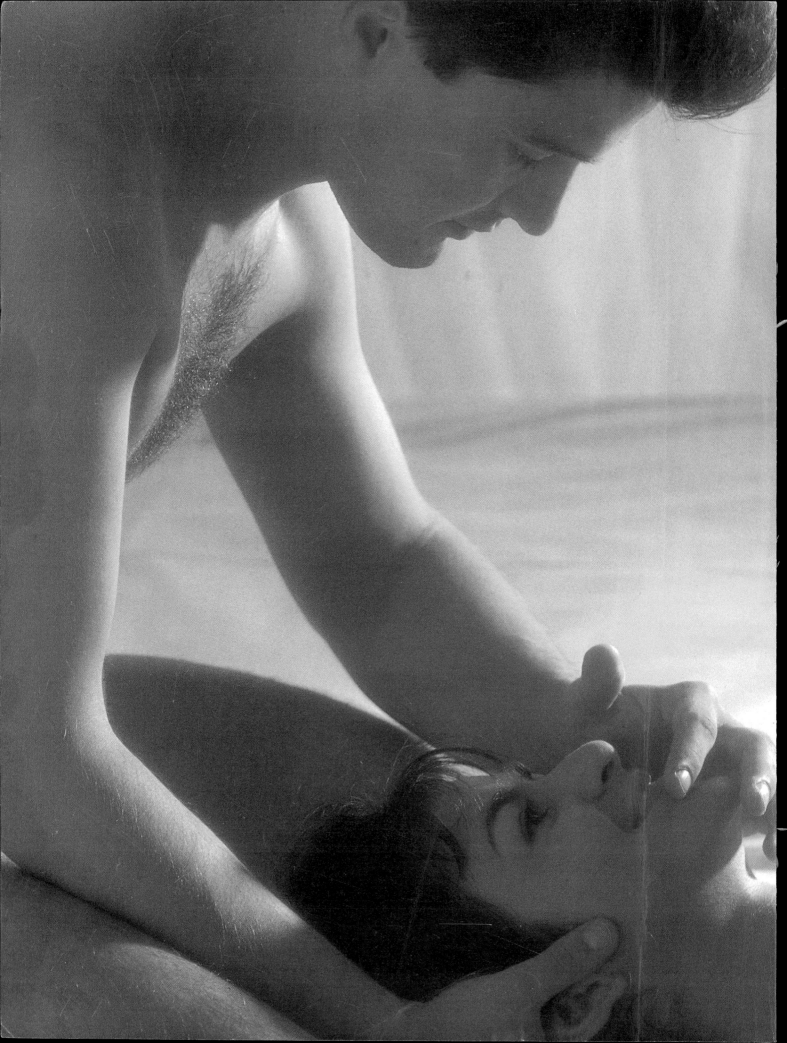

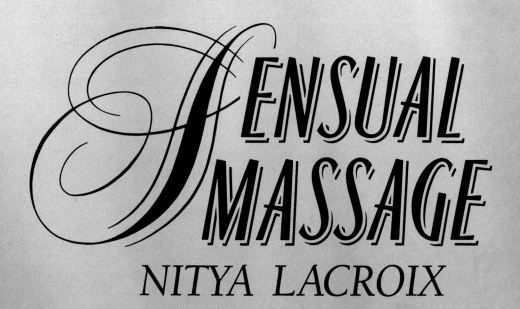

# SENSUAL MASSAGE

## NITYA LACROIX

*Photography by Antonia Deutsch*

An Owl Book
HENRY HOLT AND COMPANY
NEW YORK

*To my friends, whose encouragement, love and*
*support made this book a happy event.*

**Editor**
Carolyn Ryden

**Art editor**
Tina Vaughan

**Designers**
Laura Overton
Toni Rann

**Art director**
Anne-Marie Bulat

**Managing editor**
Daphne Razazan

Copyright © 1989 by Dorling Kindersley Limited, London
Text copyright © 1989 by Nitya Lacroix
All rights reserved, including the right to reproduce
this book or portions thereof in any form.
First published in the United States in 1990 by
Henry Holt and Company, Inc., 115 West 18th Street,
New York, New York 10011.

Library of Congress Cataloging-in-Publication Data
Lacroix, Nitya.
Sensual massage / Nitya Lacroix ; photography by Antonia Deutsch.
—1st American ed.
p.  cm.
ISBN 0-8050-1231-1 (An Owl Book: pbk.)
1. Massage.  I. Title.
RA780.5.L33  1990
615.8′22—dc20       90-4101
                          CIP

Henry Holt books are available at special discounts
for bulk purchases for sales promotions, premiums,
fund-raising, or educational use. Special editions
or book excerpts can also be created to specification.
For details contact:
Special Sales Director
Henry Holt and Company, Inc.
115 West 18th Street
New York, New York 10011

First American Edition

Recognizing the importance of preserving
the written word, Henry Holt and Company, Inc.,
by policy, prints all of its first editions
on acid-free paper.∞
3  5  7  9  10  8  6  4  2

# Contents

## Introduction
6

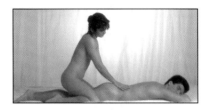

## Creating a sensual atmosphere
10

## Using oils & essences
12

## The sensitive body
14

## Sensitive hands
16

## Basic massage strokes
18

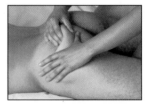

## Positions for massage
24

## Giving a sensual massage
26

*A SENSUAL MASSAGE PROGRAMME*

## Tenderness – the heart of sensual massage
28

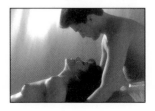

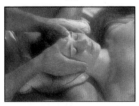
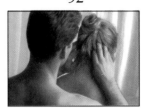
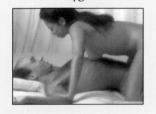
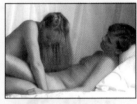
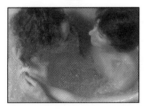
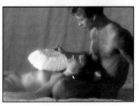
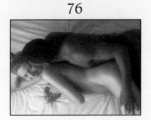

# Introduction

SENSUALITY IS THE CELEBRATION of the body and its ability for pleasure. It is an expression of ourselves through our bodies and a means of being sensitive to the needs and responses of those we love. As the art of communicating to the whole person, sensuality is the ingredient that brings spontaneity and delight to a relationship. Combined with massage, it gives us the opportunity for continuous exploration and rediscovery of the limitless capacity of the body for joy and relaxation.

### The importance of touch

Since touch has largely become taboo in Western societies, and sex is treated as a commodity, we seem to have lost our ability to celebrate our sensuality. People have become uncomfortable about touching each other as a means of sharing their more intimate and caring feelings. In fact, touch has become a forgotten language for most adults and yet it is an essential form of nourishment – a source of healing, comfort and pleasure.

Touch is the first sense we develop while still in the womb. Then at birth, touch is our first and foremost bridge with the reality that surrounds us. During childhood, a soothing caress from our parents can take away pain and hurt as if by magic. And yet once we reach adulthood, our access to receiving or giving touch is usually confined to our sexual relationships. Without the warmth imparted by touch, no matter how successful our lives may be in other areas, we are likely to feel an inner contraction and personal dissatisfaction. The sexual act itself cannot provide us with a sense of being loved, appreciated or intimate if it is our only source of close physical contact with the one we love. Indeed sensuality is as vital as sexuality in keeping a physical and emotional relationship alive and healthy.

### Touch and intimacy

In today's fast-paced world, full of pressures and stress, relationships and marriages break down at

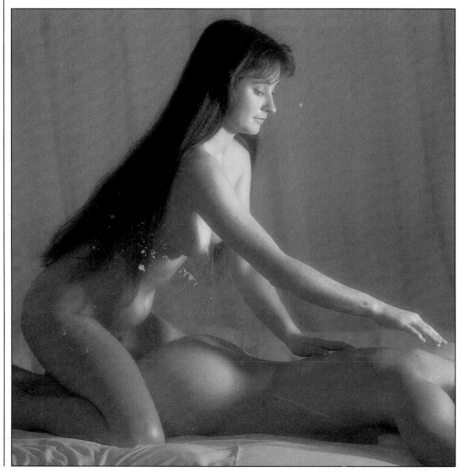

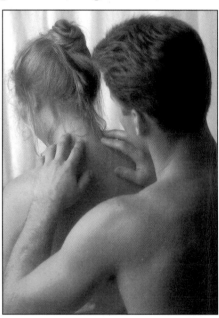

(*Above*) When you feel warm and loving towards someone, the natural response is to touch and caress.

(*Left*) Let your hands tenderly express your feelings for your partner.

(*Opposite*) The best and most relaxed massage is a silent one. But like making love, there are no rules. You may like to share endearments or even jokes.

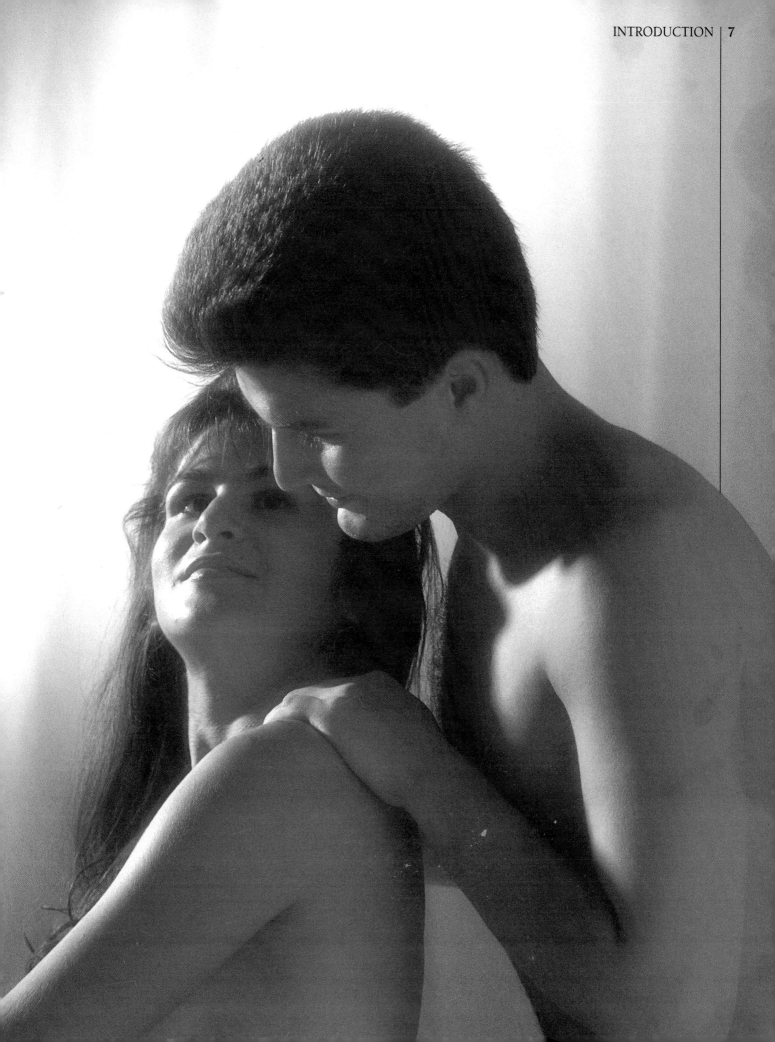

an alarming rate; after a few years many sexual relationships begin to deteriorate and lose their spontaneity. Couples grow discontent and wonder where the magic has gone. Sex becomes automatic and treated as almost a chore or a habit. Men and women begin to feel unnourished, unloved and unappreciated within their own homes and their most intimate partnerships. Increasingly, sex therapists and counsellors are stressing the value of touch and massage within relationships. They have long recognized their importance in helping couples to relax together and in overcoming difficulties with sexual intimacy.

### Exploring touch through massage

Massage is the most natural vehicle for exploring our sense of touch and enjoyment of being touched. It is a way for all of us to reach out and communicate without the barrier of words or the interference of personalities. Massage is relaxation and a means of expressing love which comes from the heart rather than the mind. Through your hands, and through your body, you can touch each other to reach not only the physical person but also mental, emotional and spiritual levels.

Massage each other on a regular basis, and you will be able to disperse the accumulated tensions that may interfere with an otherwise harmonious partnership. Your hands have the ability to return a sense of well-being both to your partner's body and to the relationship as a whole. Through touch and the way you massage, you will be able to communicate how much you value each other.

There are many ways to give a massage. A purely relaxing massage can be a deeply satisfying experience. It helps to build trust and intimacy without the immediate expectations of sexuality. At other times, within a loving partnership, massage can enrich your sexual relationship. It can take you into new and fresh dimensions of physical play and eroticism as you explore each other's sensuality together.

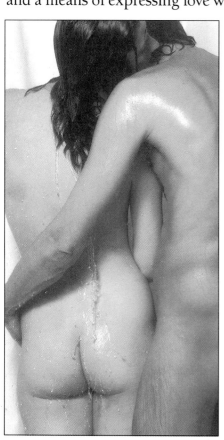

*(Above)* Take your massage into the shower for a highly sensual experience.

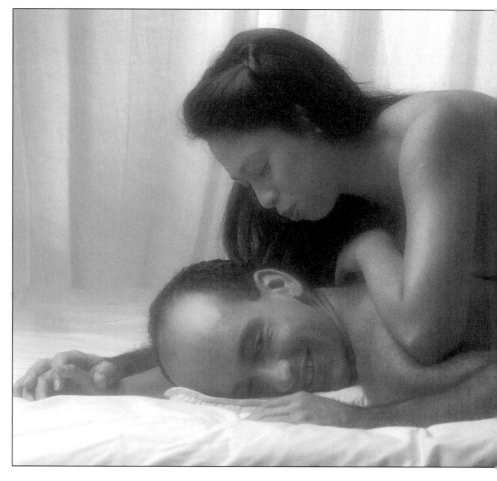

For this book, I have devised a selection of sensual massage programmes which will suit different circumstances and moods. These are intended to provide ideas, instruction and inspiration, but you should feel free to interpret them as you wish. Try to trust your hands and your own feelings. Experiment with strokes, the pressure of your touch, and the situations in which you massage. Share with each other whatever feels especially good, relaxing, stimulating and comforting. Be honest about what you do not like, and treat your massage as play not work. Once you can delight freely in the massage you are giving or receiving, this enjoyment will impart itself to your partner.

## Ground rules for a sensual massage

When you are in harmony with each other's sensuality and sexuality, there should not be any boundaries between you, but it is essential to remember that massage and touch should never be used to manipulate one another. Sensitivity to each other's needs is integral to successful massage. It is important that you never feel pressured into giving a massage. Remember that it should be an act of love genuinely proffered. If you feel too tired or reluctant to give a massage, it is better to wait for another occasion when it will seem like a celebration, not a chore.

Receiving a massage is also an art. There are few situations in life where receiving is all you have to do. This is the ultimate luxury of being given a massage. Relax and be aware that, by your receptivity, you are giving your partner the opportunity to be creative and to express his or her feelings honestly and directly through touch.

Let massage and touch become part of your lives. While you may need or want to learn some techniques, remember that it is the quality of your touch, and your presence with each other, that will deeply soothe and revitalize your bodies, heighten your pleasure and sensual awareness, and bring you closer together.

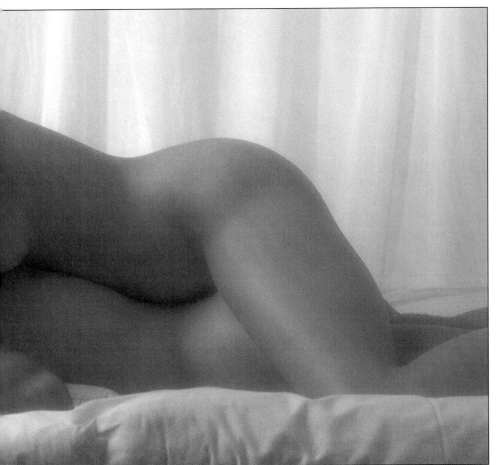

### WHEN NOT TO MASSAGE
No matter how wonderful and beneficial massage usually is, there are a few occasions when it is inadvisable. Do not massage . . .

● If your partner has a skin infection, a contagious sickness, or is running a high temperature.

● If there is severe swelling or acute inflammation affecting part of the body.

● If your partner has suffered a serious injury or has severe back pain. First consult a doctor on the proper course of treatment and ask advice on the benefits of massage.

● If your partner has thrombosis or phlebitis, and don't massage over severe varicose veins.

● If your partner is undergoing medical or psychiatric treatment of any nature. First consult your doctor on the advisability of massage.

● In any circumstances of doubt, seek medical advice before massaging.

*(Left)* The essence of sensual massage is spontaneity, expression of yourself and sensitivity to your partner.

# Creating a sensual atmosphere

WARMTH AND PRIVACY are essential ingredients for creating a sensual atmosphere for massage. Choose a place where you know you will not be interrupted, and where you can devote yourselves to each other without feeling rushed. Keep the room at a comfortable temperature (around 75°F or 24°C) throughout the massage. Body heat drops quickly when you are lying still, and a cold person soon becomes tense, which makes it difficult to relax the body through massage. Heat the room before you start, if necessary, and check that there aren't any draughts.

Wherever you decide to give the massage, make sure that the space around you is uncluttered and comfortable. You need a firm, supportive base and plenty of room to be able to move around your partner. Your bed may seem the most obvious place, but if the mattress is too soft, it will not provide essential support when you apply pressure to your strokes. It can also be difficult to move around on a bed during a massage. Instead, try placing your mattress on the floor, where there is plenty of space for movement, or use a futon, a soft rug, folded blankets, or a thick piece of foam rubber as a base for the massage.

Cover whatever surface you massage on with clean, warm sheets. Have an extra sheet or a towel close by to cover your partner, or any areas of the body you are not massaging which may start to feel cold. If you like, have a duvet or blanket handy to snuggle under in case you want to cuddle up in each other's arms at the end of the massage.

Pillows and cushions are useful for increasing support and comfort during a massage. Some people like to have a cushion under the knees when having the front of the body massaged, and just below the knees when having the back massaged. Placing a thin pillow under the base of the back, the stomach or the chest often eases tension in the body. While giving a massage, you may prefer to kneel or sit on a cushion yourself.

Have warm, dry towels ready for wiping off oil from your hands or your partner's body, especially the feet, at the end of the massage. Rubbing your partner down with a towel can be pleasurable too.

In any intimate physical contact, personal hygiene and cleanliness are very important. Taking a bath or shower together before you start is an ideal way for you both to relax and enter the mood of a sensual massage.

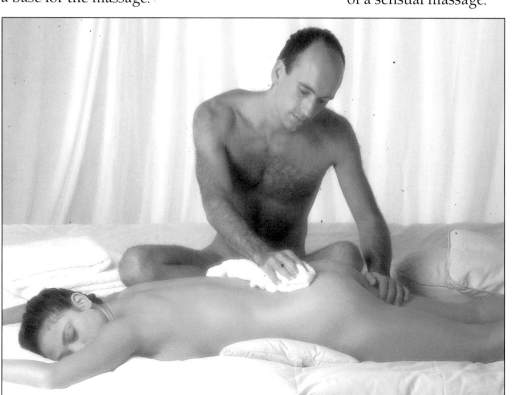

**ACCESSORIES** (*left*)
Have a few pillows and cushions nearby for comfort and support. Use towels to wipe off any excess oil and to cover any parts of your partner's body that may start to feel cold during the massage.

**MOOD** (*opposite*)
Soft, low lighting adds to a relaxing and romantic atmosphere. Music, if used, can set the mood and influence the rhythm and speed of your massage.

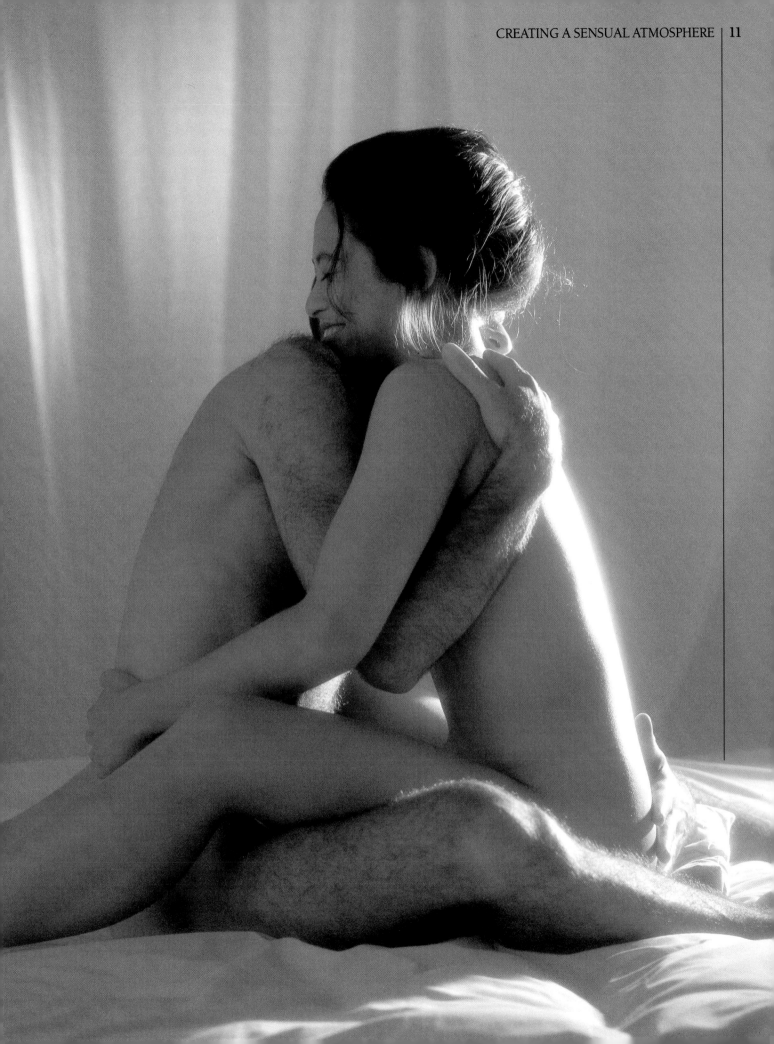

# Using oils & essences

OIL CONTRIBUTES to a smooth, flowing massage, enabling your hands to glide easily around the body. When choosing your oil, avoid those that are thick and greasy, and those with a heavy odour. Light vegetable and nut oils are easily absorbed and benefit the skin with their natural properties. Among the most popular for massage are sweet almond, avocado, grapeseed, olive, apricot kernel, peach kernel, soya and sunflower. These can be applied neat to the skin or you can add fragrant essential oils to them, using them as carrier oils, as in aromatherapy massage.

Essential oils are extracted from plants and have particular healing properties. Different essences are thought to benefit the well-being of the body, mind and emotions as well as influencing the mood of a massage. Many essential oils are also believed to have aphrodisiac qualities (see right).

A few drops of essential oil added to 25 ml (1 fl oz) of carrier oil should be sufficient for a massage, or you can add up to 25 drops of essential oil to a 50 ml (2 fl oz) bottle of carrier oil. Blended oils can go rancid after a few weeks. To help extend their shelf-life, add a teaspoonful of wheatgerm oil, which acts as an antioxidant (preservative), to your carrier oil. Only make up small amounts and store them in airtight bottles in a cool, dark place. If you choose a cheaper carrier oil such as soya, you can add a teaspoon of a more expensive, richer oil such as avocado or hazelnut, both of which are excellent for dry skins.

When massaging, keep your oil in a narrow-necked bottle with a small opening to avoid spillage and the possibility of pouring out too much at a time. Stand the bottle on a saucer and keep it within arm's reach throughout the massage. Warm the oil by rubbing each application between your hands before stroking it onto your partner's body. Cold oil will jolt the system and feels far from sensual. Apply a little oil at a time to the area you are about to massage and smooth it into the skin with a series of continuous, flowing strokes.

If your partner really does not like the feel of oil on the skin, or if you are concerned about oil stains and spills, you can use talcum powder as a substitute. However, powder does not give your hands such a smooth slide around the body, nor does it have such a sensual feel. Massage lotions are also available; these are quickly absorbed by the skin, and can be a good alternative to oil.

## APHRODISIAC OILS

The following essential oils are considered aphrodisiac. Costs of essential oils vary enormously; ylang-ylang is reasonably priced and has wonderful sensual qualities.

| | |
|---|---|
| Cedarwood | Patchouli |
| Cinnamon | Rose |
| Cloves | Sandalwood |
| Jasmine | Ylang-ylang |
| Neroli | |

## ESSENTIAL OIL BLENDS

Here are some suggestions for fragrant and therapeutic massage oil blends. As a guide, mix the drops of essential oil with 25 ml (1 fl oz) carrier oil, which should be sufficient to cover the body. The amount of oil and the number of drops will vary according to individual needs.

## AN APHRODISIAC BLEND

3 drops ylang-ylang
2 drops sandalwood
2 drops rose or jasmine
25 ml (1 fl oz) carrier oil

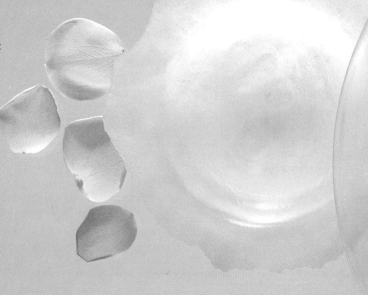

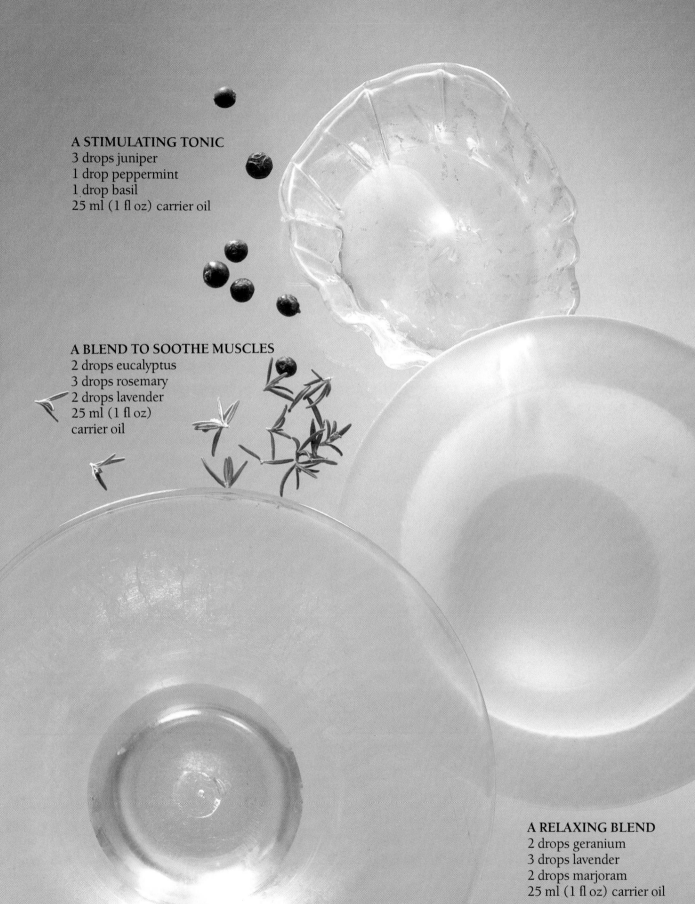

**A STIMULATING TONIC**
3 drops juniper
1 drop peppermint
1 drop basil
25 ml (1 fl oz) carrier oil

**A BLEND TO SOOTHE MUSCLES**
2 drops eucalyptus
3 drops rosemary
2 drops lavender
25 ml (1 fl oz)
carrier oil

**A RELAXING BLEND**
2 drops geranium
3 drops lavender
2 drops marjoram
25 ml (1 fl oz) carrier oil

# The sensitive body

THE WHOLE OF THE BODY is an erogenous zone capable of responding sensually and sexually to touch and stimulus. Our skin is our largest organ, vibrant with nerve endings, which receive and transmit the sensations of touching and stroking throughout the body. For this reason, massage can play a vital role in enhancing physical joy. As your hands explore the whole body, they will diffuse attention from the obvious sexual zones and start to discover the enormous potential for sensual pleasure elsewhere. From head to toe, your massage can unravel the erotic mystique of your partner's body as you realize the range of subtle and intense responses that your contact and strokes can bring.

A man, who may well believe that sexuality is genitally based, will enjoy discovering what other areas of his body can give intense physical pleasure. A woman's sexuality tends to be far less genitally focused than a man's. Her arousal may be slower,

## PLEASURE POINTS

The areas highlighted here are deliciously sensitive to being caressed, which may be because they are seldom exposed or touched lovingly.

**The lips and mouth** *are highly sensitive to touch, which enhances sensuality.*

**Stroking the lower belly** *can have a relaxing effect, heightening sexual responses and expectations.*

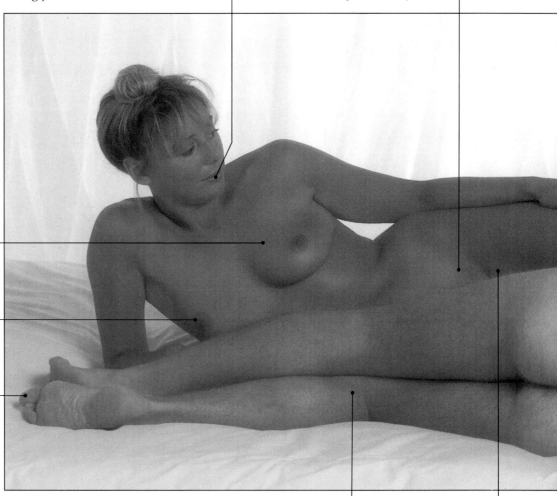

**The breasts** *give intensely pleasurable and erotic sensations when gently stroked.*

**The nipples** *respond to tender caresses, increasing feelings of sexual arousal.*

**The pad of the big toe**, *stimulated by massage, can trigger a sexual response throughout the body.*

**The back of the knee** *is exquisitely sensitive to soft stroking and gentle touching.*

**The groin**, *in close proximity to the genitals, is a highly erogenous region.*

but no less profound, and her sensual responses are heightened when care is taken to cherish and touch her entire body. Most women, and many men, respond deeply to tender caresses and all the intimate ways of physical contact that assure them they are loved for who they are.

No one appreciates being programmed for sexual response, which is why knowledge of the body's erogenous zones is worthless unless it is accompanied by a true sense of care and respect.

When you are giving a sensual massage, do not concentrate on stimulating the erogenous zones purely for effect. See the body as an integrated whole, alive to your contact and ready to transmit responses throughout its entire system. Let your touches and strokes constantly affirm your appreciation of your partner's whole body and person. In doing so, both of you can experience a deepening and expansion in the quality of your physical and emotional communication.

**The inner thighs** *can release sexual tensions when massaged, helping sensuality to flow.*

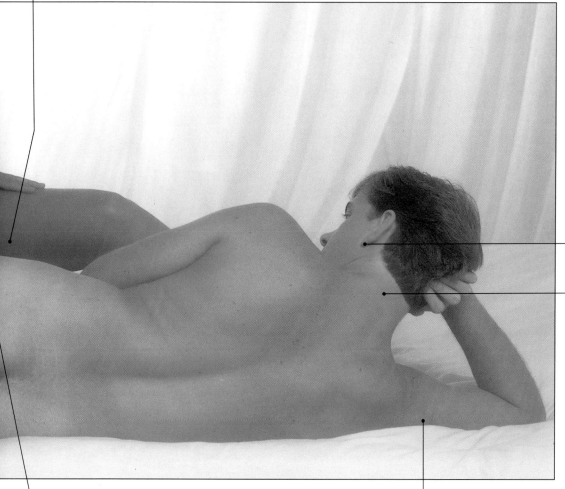

**The earlobes** *quickly transmit sensual stimuli when touched, as responses of deep pleasure.*

**Caressing the nape of the neck** *elicits strong feelings of arousal.*

**The buttocks** *are highly erogenous and respond favourably to strong, vigorous strokes.*

**The armpit** *and the soft inner arm can feel delightful when stroked gently.*

# Sensitive hands

AS YOU BEGIN TO MASSAGE, you will discover what a powerful outlet your hands are for sharing yourself and your feelings. Indeed, how you apply your hands to your partner's body during a massage is the secret of its success.

Develop your hands' sensitivity by being aware of all the sensations that they encounter each day; rough and smooth, cold and warm, soft and hard. Feel their vitality and heat by rubbing both hands together briskly for several minutes, then stopping. They will tingle as if charged with electricity. Massage your hands and exercise them frequently, to make them more supple and responsive.

When you massage someone else, let your hands yield to the body, rather than impose upon it. Imagine the hands of a potter or sculptor moulding a shape and try to bring their qualities of fluidity and

softness to your own hands. Experience for yourself the quality of your touch with this exercise. Find a warm, comfortable place to sit or lie down, undressed, and put on some music that helps you to relax and feel sensual. Think of a tiny baby's first discovery of its body and try to re-capture this sense of wonder as you let all the different areas of your hands touch, stroke and caress your entire body. Vary the effect of your strokes by moving pressure into your fingertips, thumbs and heels as you move your hands. Feel the texture of your skin and the underlying bones and muscles.

Notice all the sensations your touch creates. Through this experiment, you will come to know your hands and the many different ways in which you can use them. You will also prepare them for the time when you share their discoveries through massage with someone you love.

Each part of your hand can be used to apply a different type of stroke, pressure or effect in massage. In a single stroke you may move the emphasis from one part of your hand to another. To do this smoothly, your hands need to be soft, relaxed and flexible. The more you massage, the more attuned your hands will become to how the body feels and to what strokes it needs. You will learn to trust yourself and the ability of your hands to reassure, relax and revitalize your partner.

## THE FULL HAND

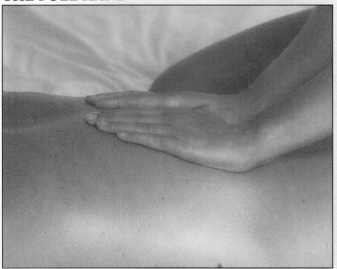

Put your full hands on the body when making smooth, flowing movements. Relax the wrists, keeping your hands soft with an even pressure. Be sure that your thumbs and fingertips also remain on the body.

## THE TIPS OF THE THUMBS

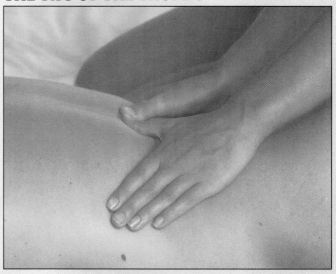

When applying pressure into a small or specific area, such as alongside the spine, you can use the tips of your thumbs. Keep the rest of your hands on the body to support the movement, but place them facing away from the thumbs.

### THE SIDES OF THE THUMBS

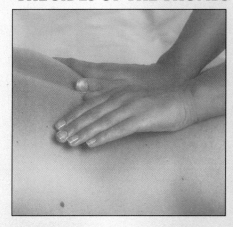

Put pressure into the sides of your thumbs and the inner edge of the heels of your hands when making circular motions. This technique is effective on the lower back, calves and feet.

### THE HEELS OF THE HANDS

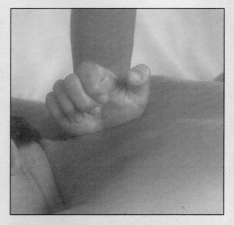

Put more pressure into the heels of your hands when you want to massage deeper into a muscle or tense areas such as around the shoulders and the base of the neck. The rest of your hands should remain relaxed.

### THE FINGERTIPS

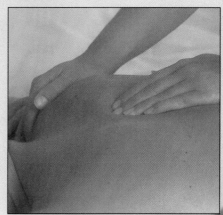

Move pressure into your fingertips by slightly cupping your palm and bending your knuckles to penetrate, stretch and relax areas of tight muscle, such as around the shoulder blades or over the upper chest.

# Basic massage strokes

THE FOLLOWING STROKES are simple to do and can be combined to make a delightful sensual massage. They will also induce an overall feeling of well-being for your partner by both relaxing and revitalizing the body, the mind and the emotions.

Start by using soft, broad, sweeping movements such as fan strokes to apply oil and help your partner to relax into the massage. Follow these with firmer, deeper massage strokes to ease tension from the body, and invigorate and stimulate the whole physical system. Build up into a rhythm with each stroke and flow from one movement into another, varying the pressure and speed of your strokes so that you both soothe and stimulate your partner's whole body. Trust your hands and your own intuition in creating your massage. The more you massage, the better and more fluid your strokes will become.

### FAN STROKES

These are a wonderful basic movement for sensual massage. Their flowing, rounded and unbroken motion makes them relaxing and unthreatening strokes on any large area of the body. They can be used throughout a massage, to relax muscles before deeper strokes, and to harmonize other strokes into the sensual mood. Fan stroking is particularly effective over the back, the chest and the legs. Lengthen or widen the stroke to suit the area you are massaging.

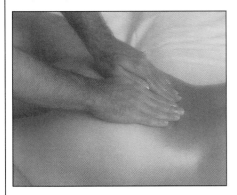

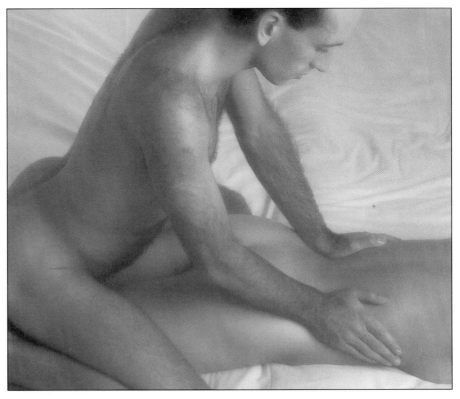

1 Place your hands side by side with your fingers close together and pointing in the direction of the stroke. Glide both hands steadily over the skin, distributing the pressure evenly across your hands.

2 When your hands have stroked as far as you wish to take them, spread them both outwards in opposite directions to make a shape like a fan, maintaining a steady pressure as you move them apart.

3 Round your stroke to complete the fan shape, and at the same time, begin to draw your hands more lightly back together as you do so. Repeat to take the stroke further up the body so that you continue to massage with a fluid movement.

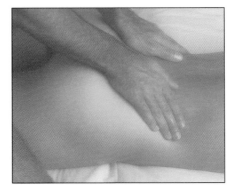

# CIRCULAR STROKES

As continuous, rounded, soothing movements, circular strokes stretch tissue and gently loosen muscles. They are sensual and relaxing, and prepare your partner for any deeper strokes that may follow. These strokes feel especially good on the back, the belly and the thighs and along the sides of the body.

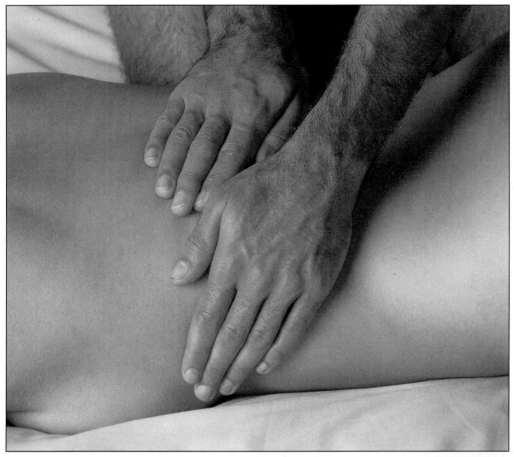

1 Lay both hands on the body, parallel but slightly apart, fingers pointing away from you. Moving from the wrist, slide both hands into a curve to start making a circle in a clockwise direction.

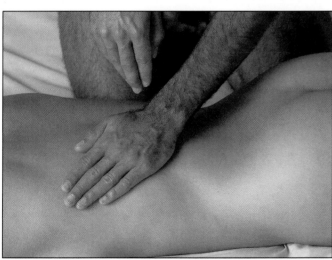

2 Lift one hand off the body after it has made a semi-circle to allow the leading hand to pass so that it can complete a full circle smoothly. In circle strokes, only one hand makes the full movement.

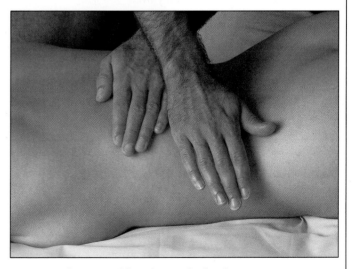

3 Pass the second hand over the leading one to return it to the body, and continue to move it so that it accentuates half of each circle traced by the leading hand. Repeat the stroke as a flowing motion.

## MILKING STROKES

These strokes are so called because of their continuous and rhythmic pulling motion on the body. Use them along the sides of the body, both from the back and the front, to relax the area around the ribs, the waist and the hips. Milking strokes also emphasize the sensual contours and curves of the body and feel pleasurably relaxing. In order to get a good pulling motion with your hands, position yourself on the opposite side of the body to the area you are going to massage so you can reach comfortably across the body's surface.

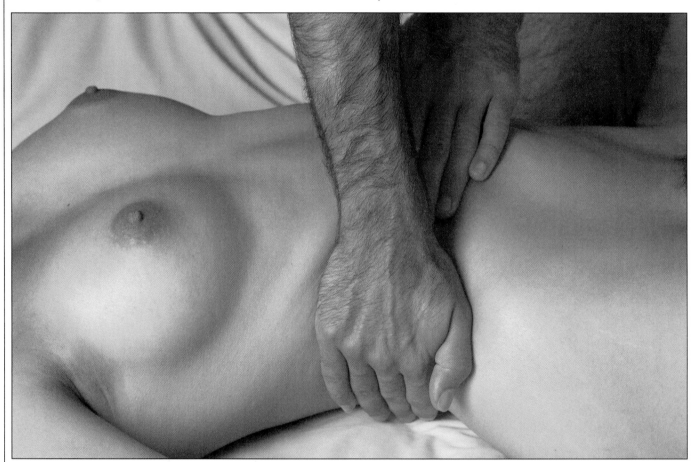

1 Place your hands over the sides of the body, slipping your fingers slightly underneath. Now pull one hand towards you, then the other, sliding the pressure from the heel to the fingertips each time.

2 As one hand reaches the centre, lift it off and replace it over the side of the body to repeat the stroke, maintaining a continuous pulling motion.

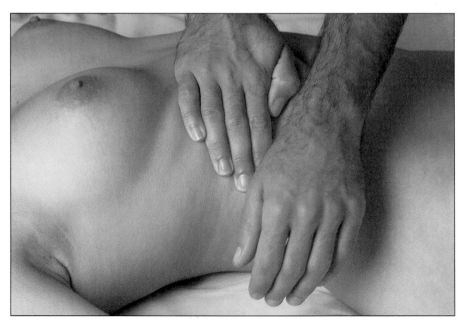

## STRETCHING

Stretches are firm, sliding movements that add a feeling of length and breadth to the body and relieve the tightness that tension creates. They can be used on the sides of the body, the legs and the back. They feel particularly good over the spine, but avoid applying too much pressure there. A variation on this movement is the diagonal stretch, where the hands move out from the centre of the spine to the shoulder and the opposite hip.

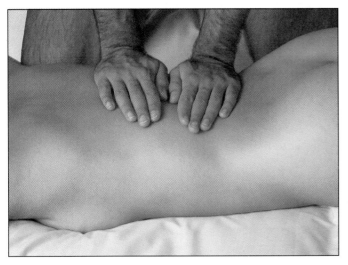

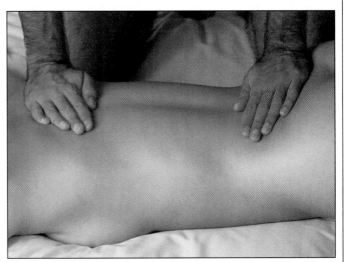

**1** Place your hands together, fingers pointing away from you, over the centre of the spine or the area that you want to release with a stretching movement.

**2** Firmly and steadily draw your hands in opposite directions. When stretching over the spine, take one hand to the top and rest the other at the base.

## RAKING STROKES

These have a delightful, releasing effect and can be applied anywhere on the body to enliven the sensory feelings of the skin. Rake over an area you have just massaged, especially after making deep and vigorous movements, to soothe and direct tension out of the body.

## FEATHER STROKES

Essential in a sensual massage, these soft brushes to the skin are soothing and playful. Linger with them over the erogenous zones, lightening your touch to skim the surface of the skin. For the not too ticklish, try a whole body massage of feather strokes for sheer pleasure.

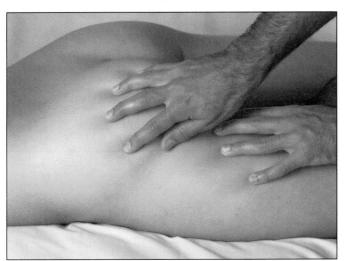

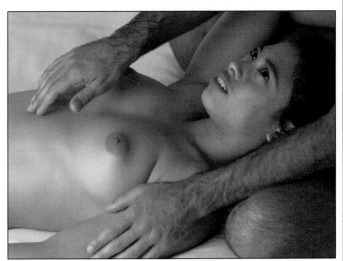

Bend your fingers so that just the tips rest on the skin and make short, firm movements down or out of the body. This stroke feels good on the arms and legs after they have been relaxed with soothing strokes. Use both hands together or let one hand follow the other.

Delicately trace your fingertips over the skin, using one hand after the other in a continuous movement, or lingering playfully with just one hand at a time. Change the pressure and speed of your strokes slightly to vary the sensations of your touch.

# Deeper strokes

ASENSUAL MASSAGE is focused on pleasure and relaxing and arousing the body. It is not specifically concerned with tension areas or the need to correct them. However, few of us are without tension, particularly in the neck, shoulders and lower back, so we often appreciate deeper massage in these regions. The broad, sweeping and relaxing movements of sensual massage are a gentle and loving way to prepare your partner's body for deeper and more invigorating strokes.

## FLESH KNEADING

This form of kneading rolls the flesh between the fingers and thumb of each hand. Its rhythmic motion loosens the underlying muscles and the stroke feels especially relaxing on fleshy areas such as the thighs and buttocks. It is very relaxing for breaking down tension in specific areas such as around the shoulders and the base of the neck.

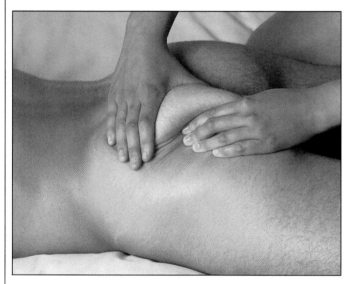

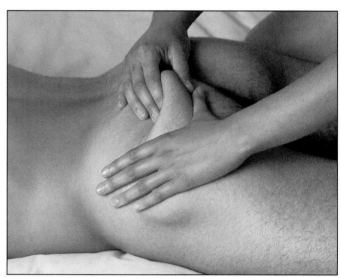

1 Lift, roll and press the flesh by moving the pressure between the fingers and thumb of one hand in a squeeze-release motion.

2 Alternate the movement rhythmically with the other hand to produce a continuous wave-like motion between the fingers and thumb of each hand.

## BROAD KNEADING

Apply pressure from the heels of the hands and the sides of the thumbs while making this stroke.

## THUMB PAD KNEADING

Ideal for deeper penetration over thick muscles, fleshy areas, and muscle attachments.

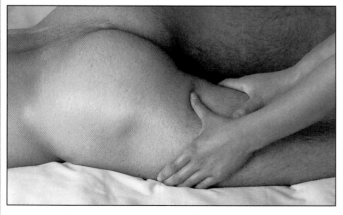

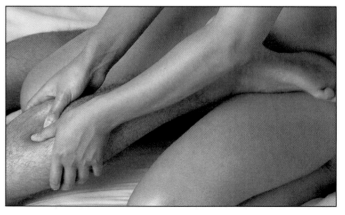

Move your hands in continuous alternate circular motions, putting pressure on the first half of each circle and lessening it on the return.

Rotate your thumbs alternately in opposing moving circles. Apply pressure from the thumb pads, using the rest of the hands as support as you make the stroke.

## FINGERTIP ROTATION

A perfect stroke for around and under muscle attachments and bony areas such as elbows and knees, as well as small tension points such as the base of the skull. Apply on areas already relaxed by softer strokes.

## HEEL OF HAND ROTATION

The heels of the hands are excellent for applying pressure for deeper massage and loosening muscles.

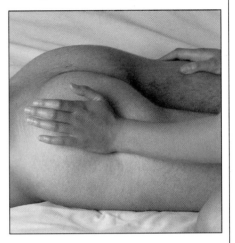

Use just the heel with the rest of the hand raised and relaxed. Keep your arm and elbow loose and your wrist softly flexed. Rotate the heel into the muscle, applying pressure on the upper half of each circle and returning more lightly.

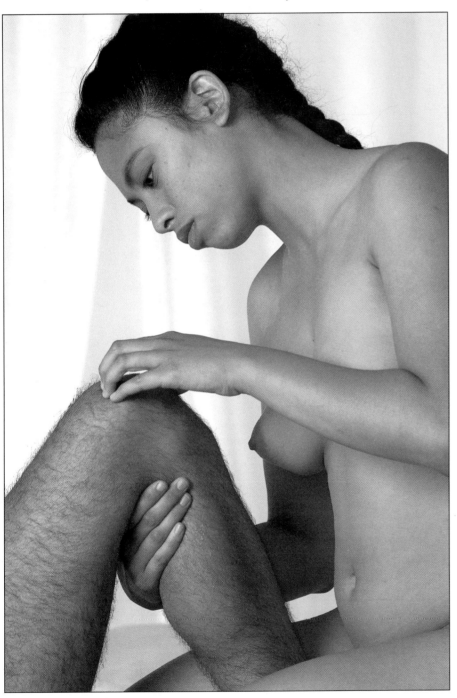

Keeping your knuckles slightly bent and your wrist flexible, use the fingertips of one hand to apply pressure in small circular movements. While using one hand, always keep the other hand on the body as support. The motion is spiral, moving forwards slowly so that the muscle preceding the stroke begins to relax before penetration. Increase the pressure in your fingertips as you feel the tissue relaxing underneath.

# Positions for massage

WHEN YOU MASSAGE someone you love, it is natural to focus your concern on how relaxed and comfortable he or she is. However, it is just as important to take care of yourself while giving a massage. The more relaxed you are, the more you will enjoy what you are doing, and the better the massage will be. If you finish a massage feeling tired or physically strained, you may feel resentful about giving a massage again.

Your partner should lie on a surface firm enough to support your movements and your weight. Throughout your massage, take note of how your own body is feeling and keep relaxing any tense areas. Have an image of your spine as being elongated as you move into your strokes. Your shoulders should feel relaxed and wide, not tense and tight, and your neck and head should feel loose and easy.

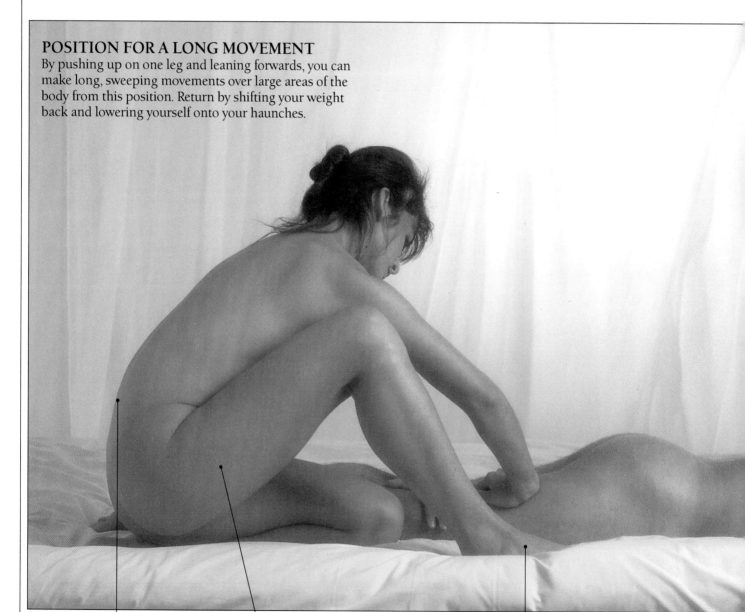

**POSITION FOR A LONG MOVEMENT**
By pushing up on one leg and leaning forwards, you can make long, sweeping movements over large areas of the body from this position. Return by shifting your weight back and lowering yourself onto your haunches.

**Keep your spine** *loose and stretched.*

**To raise your body** *and lean forwards, shift your balance from your haunches to your lower leg.*

**Put your weight** *onto your foot to push yourself forwards.*

Change your position when necessary so you always face towards your strokes – don't twist your body into uncomfortable positions – and avoid putting strain on your back at all times. To lean forwards or backwards, tilt your body at the pelvis and hips rather than bending your shoulders. Be aware of your legs and feet, and let them help to support your weight when necessary. Here are some helpful positions to use as you massage.

## STRADDLING

An intimate position that allows you to lean into your strokes with even pressure.

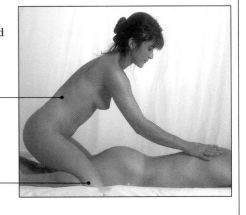

**Keep your body raised** *slightly to avoid lowering your full weight onto your partner.*

**Use your knees** *and lower leg muscles to support you.*

## SITTING

This is a good position when you are massaging small areas of the body like the feet and the face, and the belly.

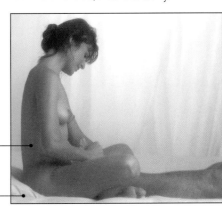

**Sit comfortably** *with your legs crossed and your back loose and straight.*

**Sit on the edge** *of a cushion to help tip your pelvis forwards.*

## KNEELING

A good position for most massage strokes. To reach further, lean forwards from your hips and knees. Move into the position shown on the left to cover a larger area.

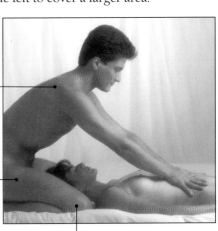

**Keep the upper half** *of your body lengthened and relaxed as you massage.*

**For a longer reach,** *lean forwards from your hips and knees.*

**Set your knees apart** *so your body feels balanced.*

**Your partner** *should feel comfortable and relaxed.*

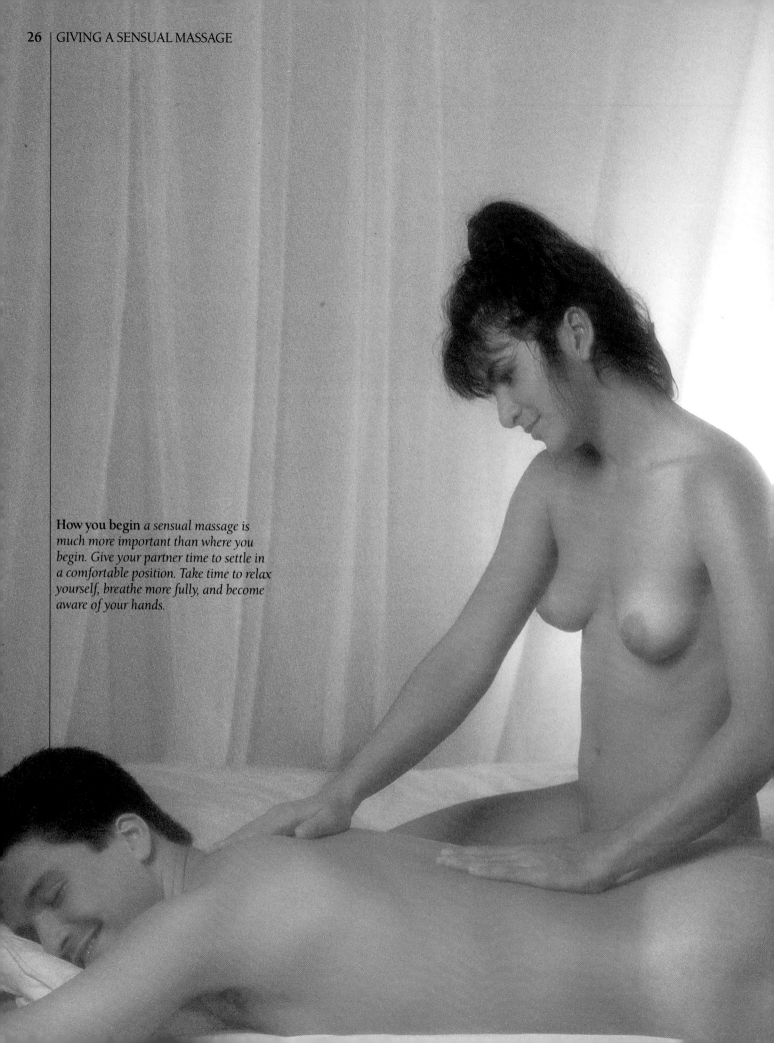

**How you begin** *a sensual massage is much more important than where you begin. Give your partner time to settle in a comfortable position. Take time to relax yourself, breathe more fully, and become aware of your hands.*

# Giving a sensual massage

THE FIRST TOUCH of a massage is the most significant as it sets the mood for the whole massage. Start by simply resting your hands gently on your partner's body for a few moments, giving them time to melt into the contact of touch. Having settled into this initial contact, you can begin to apply the oil. Don't pour cold oil directly onto your partner, tip a few drops onto the palm of one hand first, then rub both palms together to warm and coat them with the oil. Now spread the oil, but only over the part of the body you are about to massage; oily skin quickly becomes cold and sticky. Put enough oil on your hands so that your strokes are smooth and flowing. Too much oil makes a massage messy and awkward, and also prevents your hands having real contact with your partner's body.

Having made contact, try not to break it until you finish your massage. If you remove your hands to re-apply oil, allow another part of your body, such as your leg or your arm, to touch your partner. When you need to change your position, do so with full awareness of your partner's body. Avoid making any abrupt moves as they will break the smooth flow of the massage.

Rhythm is important in your strokes. Move fluidly between soft and deep, and slow and fast, strokes. Throughout the massage, treat the body as a whole, stroking from one area to another with flowing continuity. As no stroke feels complete if it is broken or ended suddenly, round off each one in a circular motion if it changes direction or passes over a curve such as a hip or a shoulder. Alternatively, strokes can be extended right out of the body via the neck and head, arms or legs.

Finish your massage as sensitively as you began, withdrawing your hands slowly from your partner's body. Be patient and aware of whatever expectations have arisen; now is the time to be sensitive and respectful to each other's mood. Making love may be the natural outcome to sensual massage, but so too could rest, sleep or conversation.

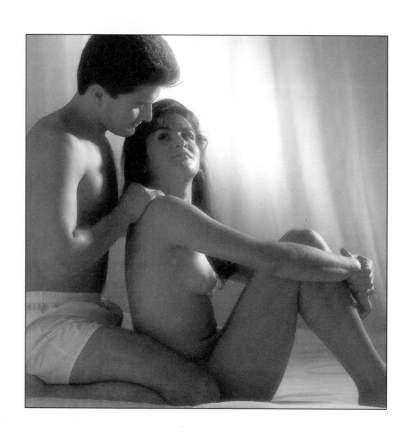

# Tenderness – the heart of sensual massage

THE VERY ESSENCE of a sensual massage is the element of care and tenderness in your touch. Through it, you communicate your deepest and most intimate feelings for your partner in a more immediate way than you may be able to in words.

In this massage programme, the sequence of strokes over the upper body covers some of its most vulnerable and sensitive areas. The chest often stores emotional feelings of love, sadness and joy. The contact of your hands over this area can impart feelings of comfort and serenity, and bring emotional release and relaxation as you encourage your partner to let go completely into your care. The breasts and face are such intimate parts of the body that they invite only the most sincere and gentle touches. When you caress the body of someone you love, do so with reverence. Let your hands express how much you value that person's presence in your life.

# The opening caress...

KNEEL AT YOUR PARTNER'S HEAD and rest it between your knees on a thin cushion. Open the massage with a large, flowing stroke, sweeping over the chest, the rib-cage, around the shoulders and up out of the neck and head. Sensual and fluid, it not only emphasizes the shape of the upper body but also helps it to relax by opening the chest for deeper breathing and the release of emotional feelings. Spread the oil as you make this stroke and repeat it until you feel the area soften and relax under your hands.

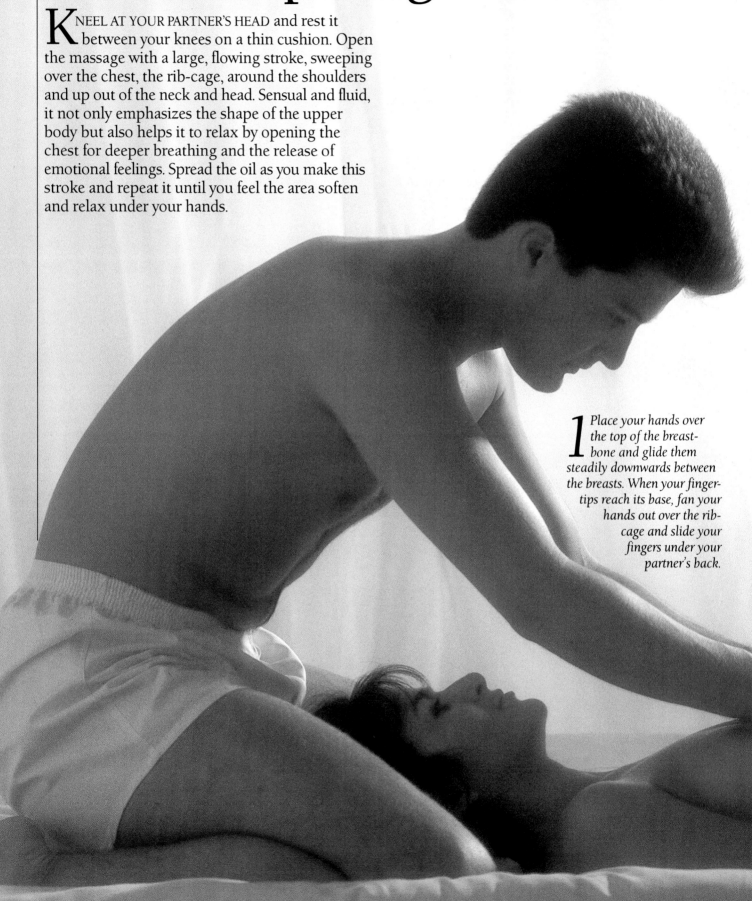

*1 Place your hands over the top of the breast-bone and glide them steadily downwards between the breasts. When your finger-tips reach its base, fan your hands out over the rib-cage and slide your fingers under your partner's back.*

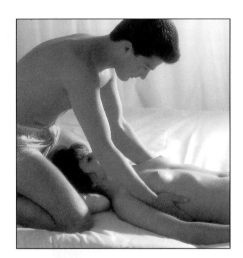

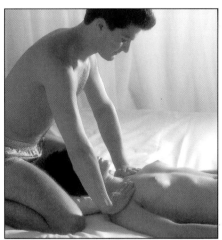

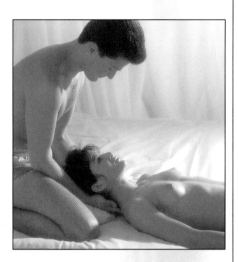

**2** *Moulding your hands around your partner's body, pull upwards along the sides of her ribs in a stretching motion. This stretching movement will bring a sense of length and release to the upper body, which feels wonderful.*

**3** *When your hands reach the armpits, turn your wrists once to swing the heels of your hands onto the chest and then outwards towards the shoulders. Add pressure first to the heels and then to the fingers as you glide them towards the shoulders, stretching and relaxing the muscles below the collar-bone and across the upper chest.*

**4** *Sweep your hands around the shoulders, pulling the heels up into the muscles behind. Rest your fingers on each side of the spine to let your partner's neck relax into the warm support of your hands. Draw them firmly up the neck, lifting the head slightly as you reach the hairline, then run your fingers out through her hair.*

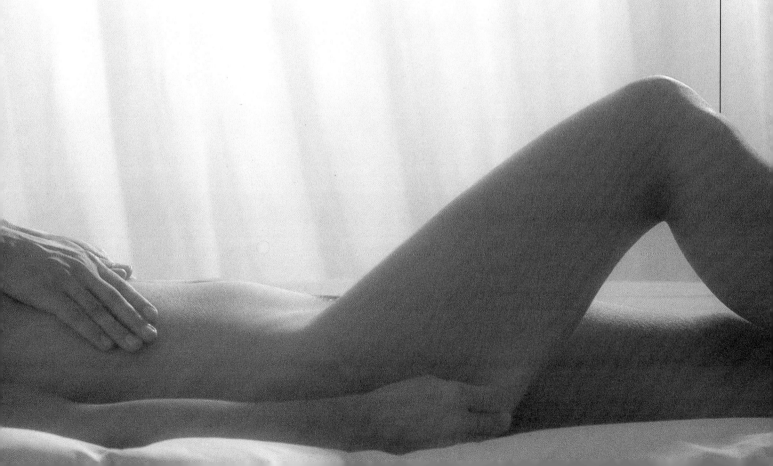

# Relaxing play...

ENCOURAGE YOUR PARTNER to relax fully by
letting you take charge of her body. Create a
releasing effect through the chest and shoulders
by stretching and lifting her body. To accomplish
this stroke successfully, be aware of your own body
position. Keep your whole back
lengthened, using the lower part of your
body to support your movement. However,
do not try this if your partner is a lot
heavier than you as it could put a strain
on your own back.

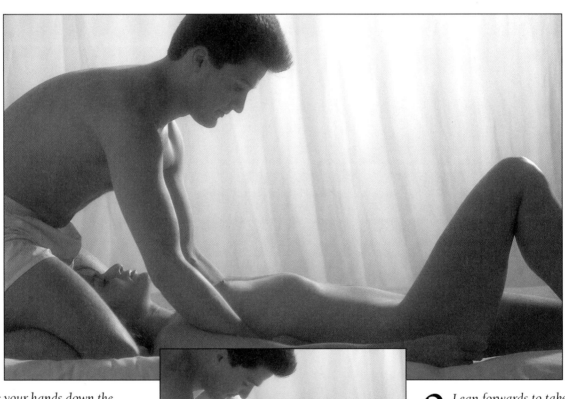

**1** *Glide your hands down the
breastbone and over the base of
the ribs, then slide them under
your partner's back with your fingers
pointing inwards and thumbs facing
down. Using your body weight, pull
your hands up the back to lift the chest
and rib-cage slightly off the mattress.
When you reach the armpits, slide your
hands onto the chest, over the
shoulders and down the arms.*

**2** *Lean forwards to take her wrists
in your hands and slowly lift
her arms, rising up on your
knees. Once the arms are straight, pull
gently upwards to stretch around the
shoulder joints. Now slowly lower her
arms, first from the shoulders to the
elbows, then from the elbows to the
wrists, so that they are spread wide
and above her shoulders with her
hands fully relaxed.*

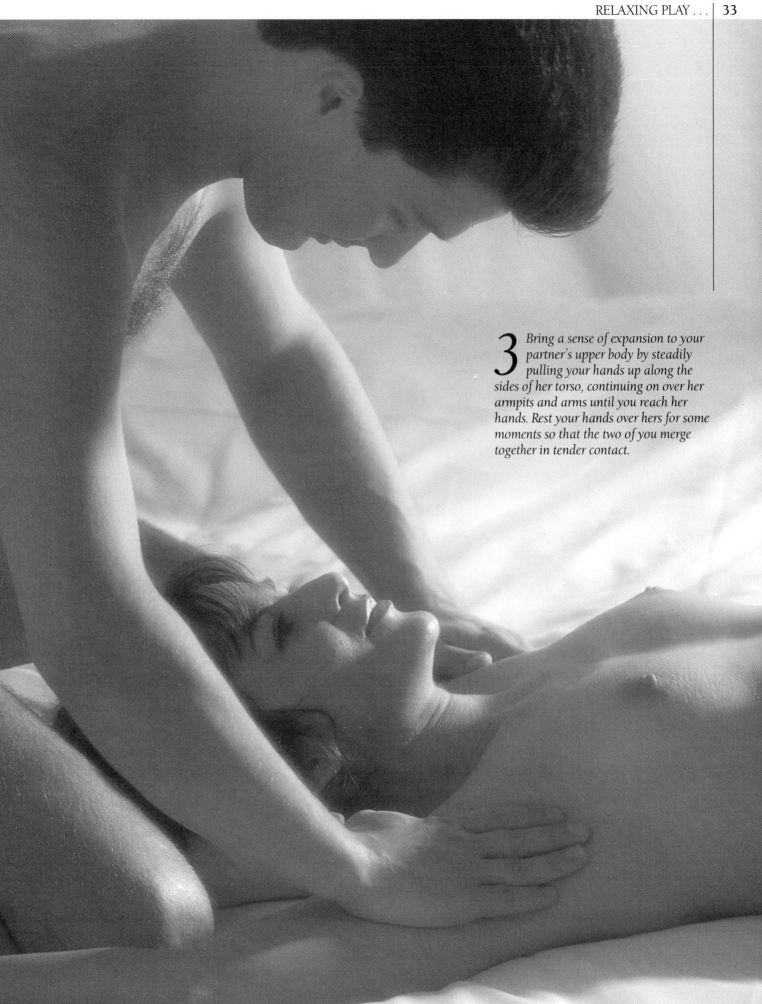

3 Bring a sense of expansion to your partner's upper body by steadily pulling your hands up along the sides of her torso, continuing on over her armpits and arms until you reach her hands. Rest your hands over hers for some moments so that the two of you merge together in tender contact.

# Teasing & enchanting ...

**1** *Playfully tease and enchant your partner by leaning forwards over her body, being careful not to press on her hair or face, and planting soft, intimate kisses delicately over her belly.*

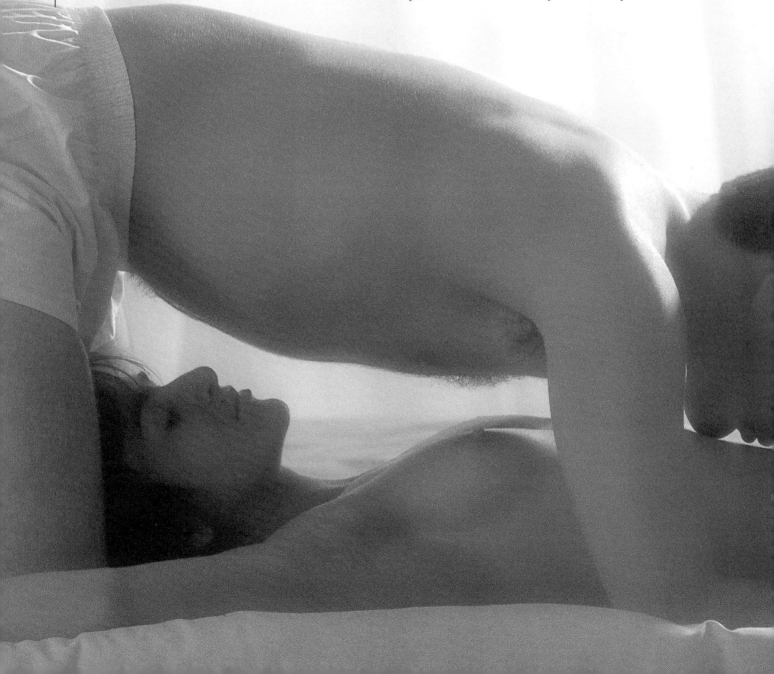

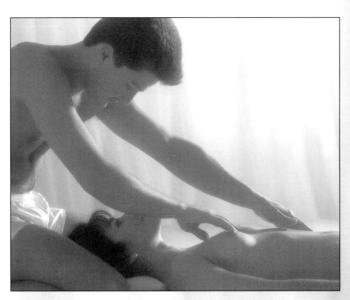

**2** *Trace your fingers in light feather strokes up from her belly and over her breastbone, upper chest and shoulders, enlivening her skin with the soft brush of your fingertips. Continue the strokes out over her neck and head, gently combing your fingers out through her hair.*

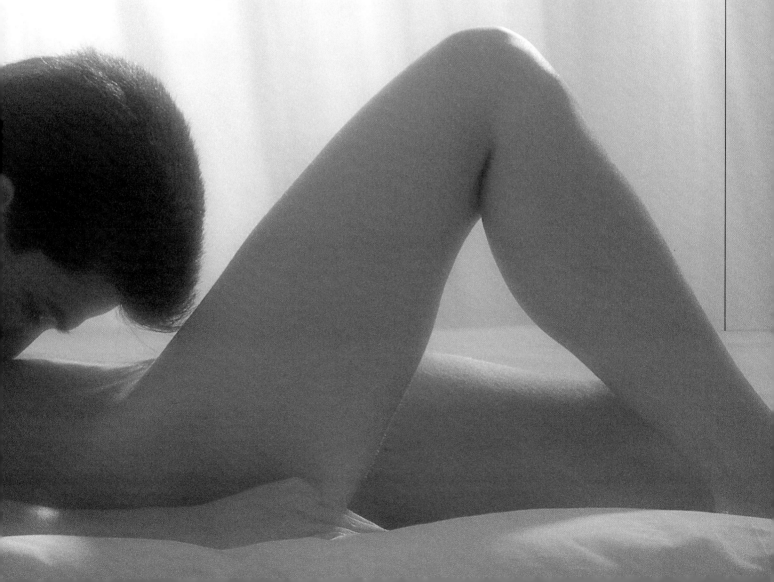

# Caressing the breasts...

A WOMAN'S BREASTS are highly sensitive and erogenous. Her relationship to this feminine area of her body will reflect her deepest feelings towards herself as a woman.

Always touch the breasts with respect and tenderness. Be sensitive to your partner's feelings. In massage, it is important to remember that the breasts are glands, not muscles, and should never have any pressure applied to them.

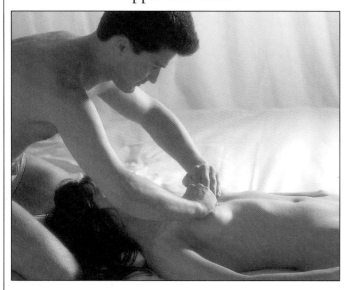

*1 Create a feeling of space around the breasts by placing the fingertips of both hands together at the centre of the base of the breastbone. Draw your fingertips outwards, stretching in short horizontal lines, working steadily upwards. Do not work over the breasts themselves. (On a man, this stroke can be taken right over each side of the rib-cage to relax the tissue between the ribs.)*

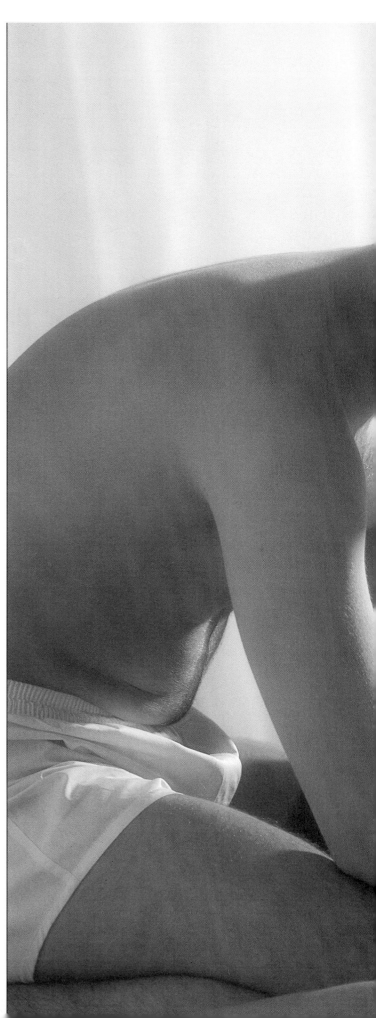

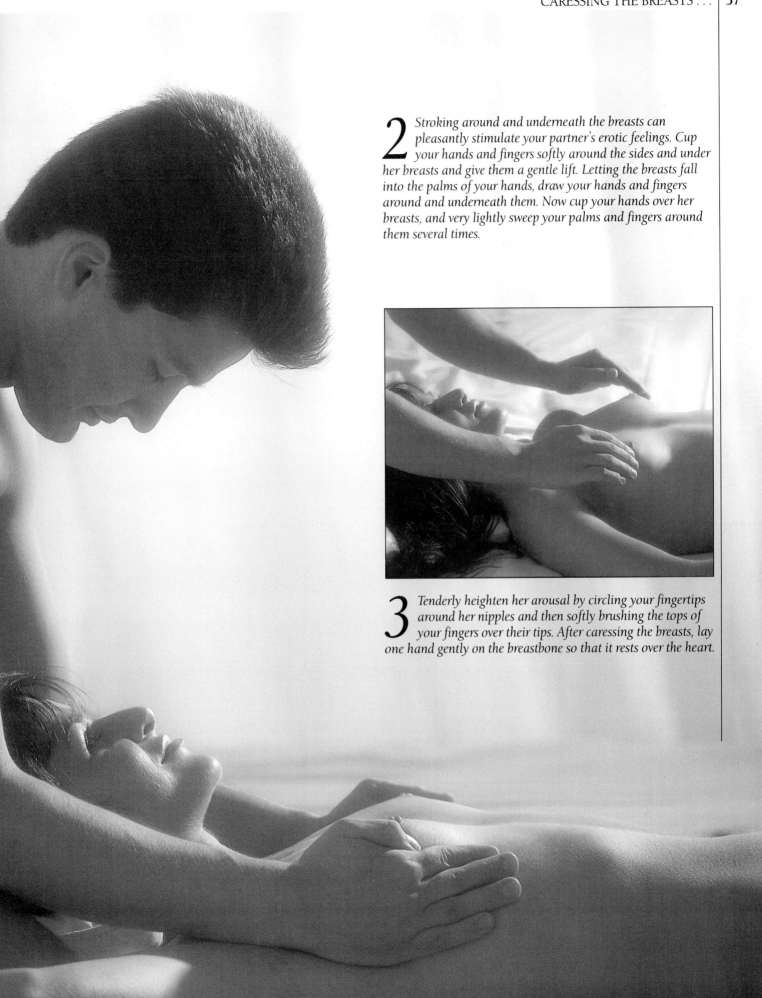

2 Stroking around and underneath the breasts can pleasantly stimulate your partner's erotic feelings. Cup your hands and fingers softly around the sides and under her breasts and give them a gentle lift. Letting the breasts fall into the palms of your hands, draw your hands and fingers around and underneath them. Now cup your hands over her breasts, and very lightly sweep your palms and fingers around them several times.

3 Tenderly heighten her arousal by circling your fingertips around her nipples and then softly brushing the tops of your fingers over their tips. After caressing the breasts, lay one hand gently on the breastbone so that it rests over the heart.

# Cherishing touches...

LIGHTLY STROKE UP from your partner's breasts to her neck and throat, which are also highly sensitive and sensually responsive. Delight your partner by tracing your fingers softly over the front of the throat up towards her chin before you start to massage her face. Gently outline her features with your hands and fingertips, easing away tension from her jaw, touching delicately over her cheek-bones and eyes, and relaxing her forehead and temples. Linger playfully over her lips and ears with sensual, teasing strokes that can excite and enrapture your partner.

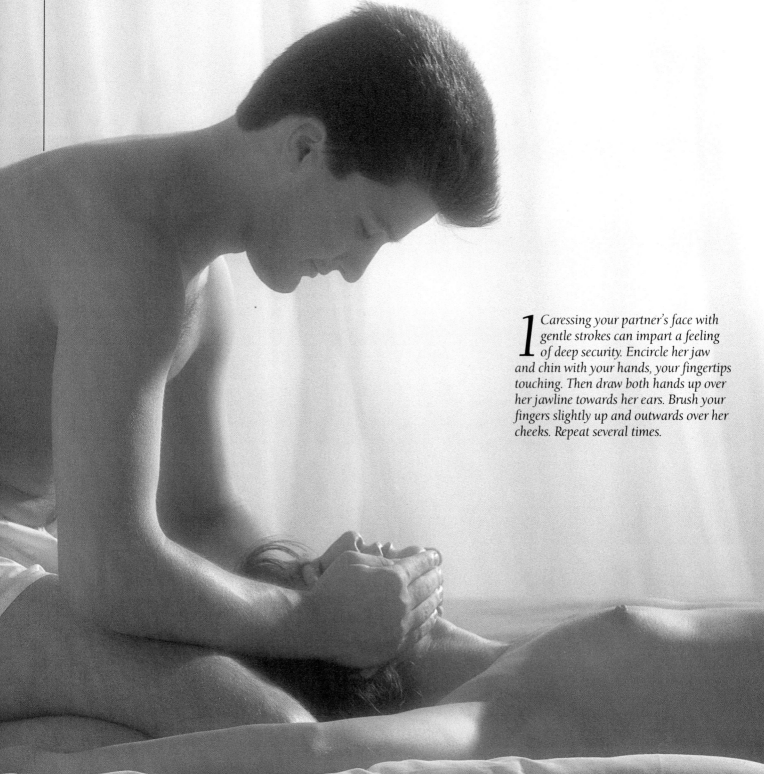

*1 Caressing your partner's face with gentle strokes can impart a feeling of deep security. Encircle her jaw and chin with your hands, your fingertips touching. Then draw both hands up over her jawline towards her ears. Brush your fingers slightly up and outwards over her cheeks. Repeat several times.*

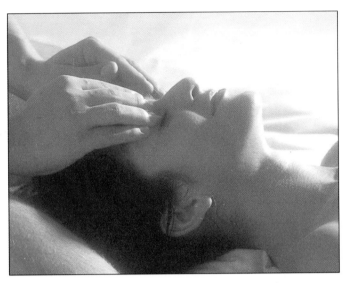

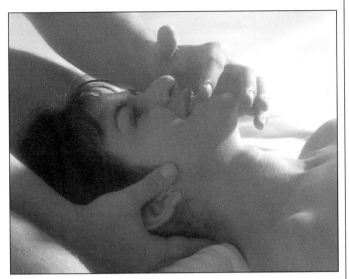

2 Trace your fingertips over the cheek-bones, under the eyes, softly over the eyelids and across the eyebrows, always moving outwards and following the structure of the bones. Make your strokes smooth and consistent, covering both sides of the face at one time. Soothe away all anxiety from the forehead with gentle sweeps of your fingers from the centre, out over the temples and into the hair. Repeat these strokes several times to relax your partner fully.

3 Delicately trace the shape of your partner's mouth with your fingertip, gently stroking around and over her lips slowly several times. Make your touches as light and soft as you can. Slip your finger onto the sensitive surface just inside your partner's lips and glide it over the soft, moist skin.

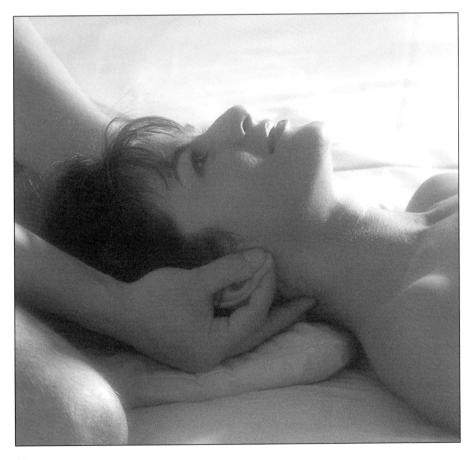

4 Touching or kissing the ears can readily enflame sexual feelings. Support the underside of the ears with your fingertips and begin to massage all over the lobes and the outer ears, making tiny rotations with your thumbs. Gently run your fingers around the inside of each ear, but do not push down into the ear canal. Now stroke lightly up and down and around the back of the ears. Finish the massage with tender strokes over the head and out through her hair.

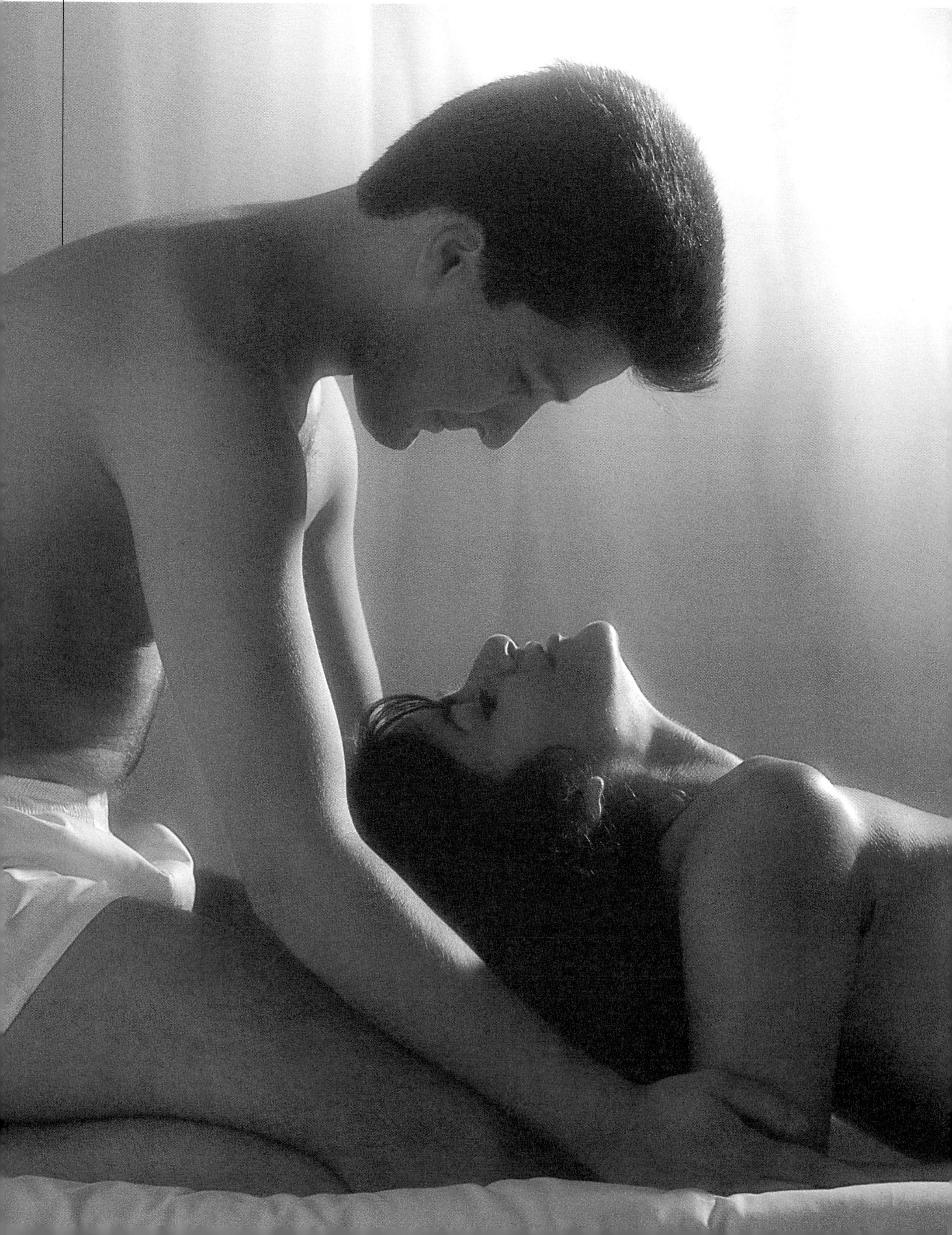

*A sensual massage within an intimate relationship has more to do with love than technique.
By the very nature of your loving touch, your partner will relax deeply and feel emotionally and physically cherished . . .*

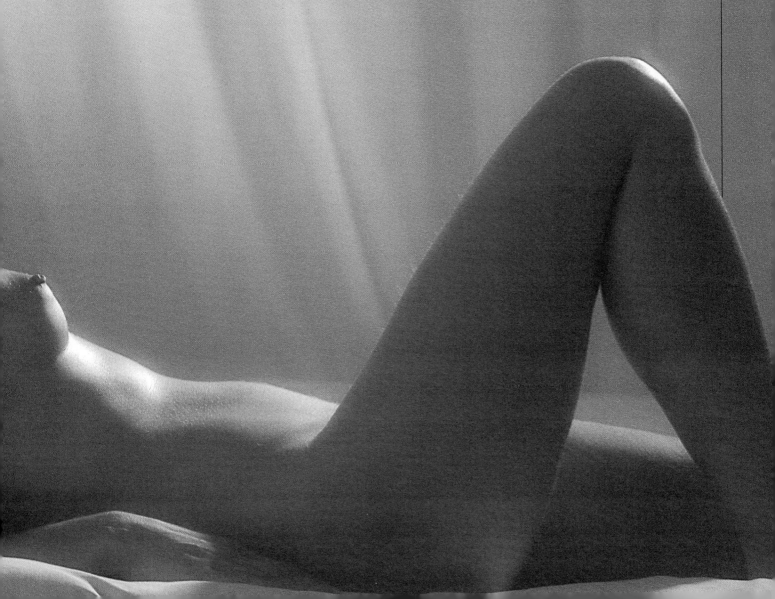

# Neck & head massage

EVERYONE APPRECIATES a neck and head massage as it helps to release all the tensions that so often accumulate in this area. These can be hard to dispel, preventing spontaneity and total relaxation. A stiff neck is also a common cause of enervating headaches, but a gentle massage over the neck can soon melt such pain away. Avoid trying to penetrate tight muscles too quickly as this can cause more discomfort. Don't apply pressure on the front of the neck as this will feel uncomfortable and threatening to your partner, whereas soft strokes here feel good.

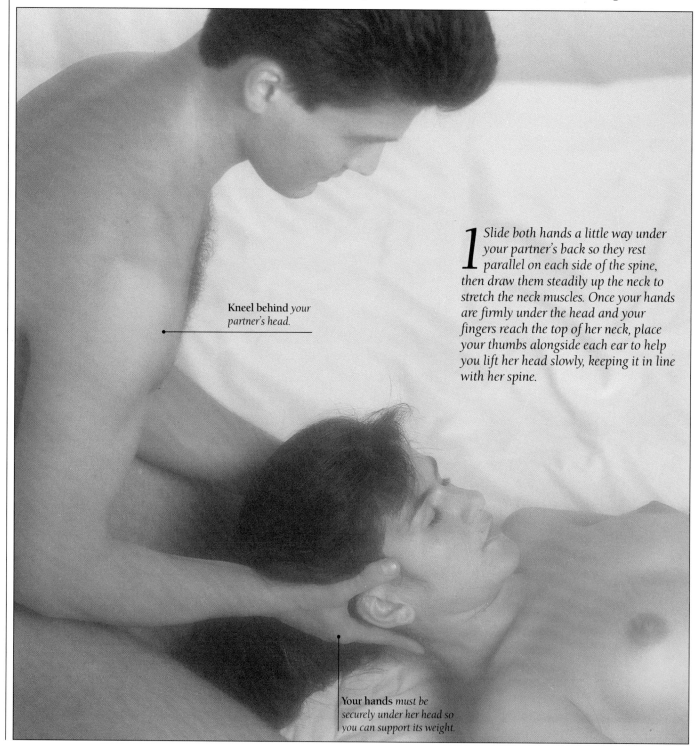

Kneel behind *your partner's head.*

*1 Slide both hands a little way under your partner's back so they rest parallel on each side of the spine, then draw them steadily up the neck to stretch the neck muscles. Once your hands are firmly under the head and your fingers reach the top of her neck, place your thumbs alongside each ear to help you lift her head slowly, keeping it in line with her spine.*

**Your hands** *must be securely under her head so you can support its weight.*

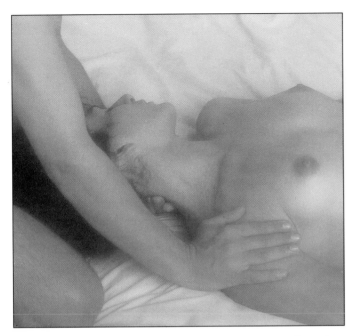

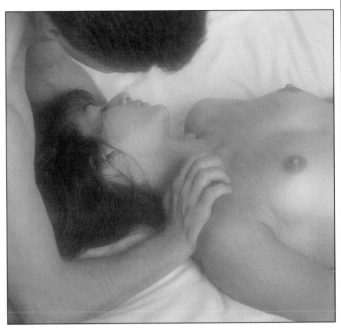

**2** Turn the head to one side and let it rest against the palm of one hand, lightly gripping the back of the neck with your fingers. Create a releasing stretch down the side of the neck into the shoulder by pressing down on the exposed shoulder with your free hand. Release the pressure from here slowly to help the muscles relax.

**3** Stroke down the side of the neck and into the muscle behind the shoulder, putting pressure into the heel of your hand. When you reach the shoulder bone, turn your wrist and soften your hand as you sweep it around the shoulder and then glide it up the back of the neck. Repeat over the muscles running down the side of the neck.

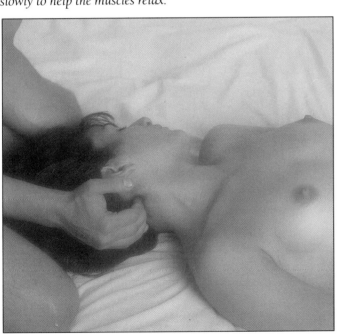

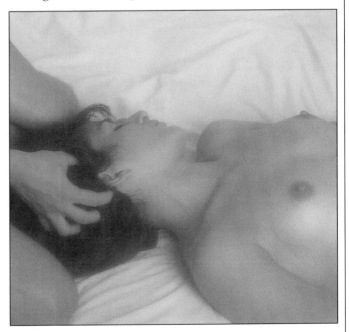

**4** Help free the area directly under the base of the skull by applying pressure with your fingertips and making small circular movements just under the bone. Work these rotations from the top of the spine out towards the back of the ear. Be firm but sensitive with your touch, deepening the pressure only as you feel the muscles relax.

**5** Work your fingertips in circular motions over the scalp as if shampooing your partner's hair; move from the base of the skull to the crown. Turn your partner's head and repeat all these strokes on the other side of her neck and head. Finish by resting the head so that it is comfortable and aligned with her spine.

# Face massage

HAVING YOUR FACE TOUCHED is a very personal and intimate experience. Be sensitively aware of your hands and especially your fingers when you give this massage. Use a firm, steady and tender touch, and direct your strokes outwards over the skin. Don't stroke around the face at random as this can be irritating and uncomfortable. Let the features and bone structure of your partner's face be your natural guide.

**Kneel or sit** *behind your partner's head.*

1 *Cradle your partner's head between your hands, placing them evenly around its crown with your thumbs resting downwards on her forehead. Hold her head for some moments and then slowly draw your hands away, stroking up through the hair and over the scalp as if brushing away the day's tension.*

**Ensure that** *your partner's head and neck are relaxed and comfortable. Let her rest her head on a thin cushion if this helps.*

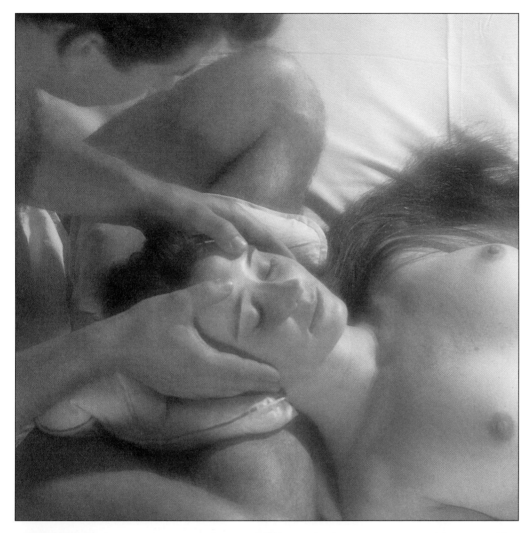

**2** *Rest your fingers around her face and place your thumbs on the centre of her forehead and brow. Slide them firmly outwards towards the temples. Repeat the stroke several times until you have covered the entire forehead, and complete each movement by sweeping your thumbs around the temples.*

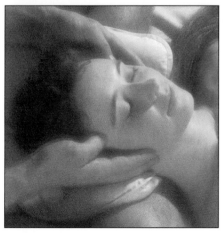

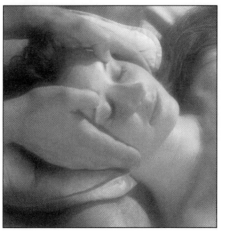

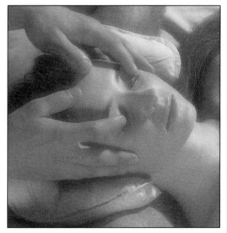

**3** *Slide your thumbs steadily around the temples several times. This stroke has an extremely soothing effect and helps to release the tension that gathers across the forehead and scalp and behind the eyes.*

**4** *Position your thumb tips on the inner edge of the eyebrows and draw them out steadily under the brow bone from the inner to the outer edges. Continue to rest your hands softly against your partner's head.*

**5** *Provided your partner isn't wearing contact lenses, increase the feelings of tenderness by lightly and gently stroking with your fingertips over her closed eyelids. Then rest your hands softly over her eyes for a few moments.* ▷

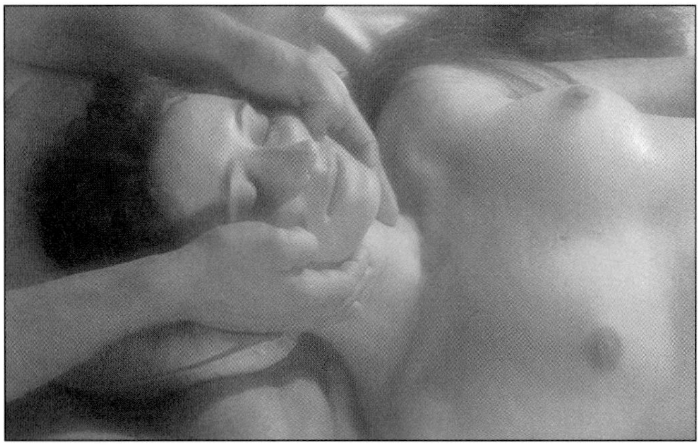

6 *Place your thumbs on the bridge of your partner's nose and run them steadily down each side of it, then move them outwards under her cheek-bones. Repeat several times, sweeping your hands out through her hair before returning them.*

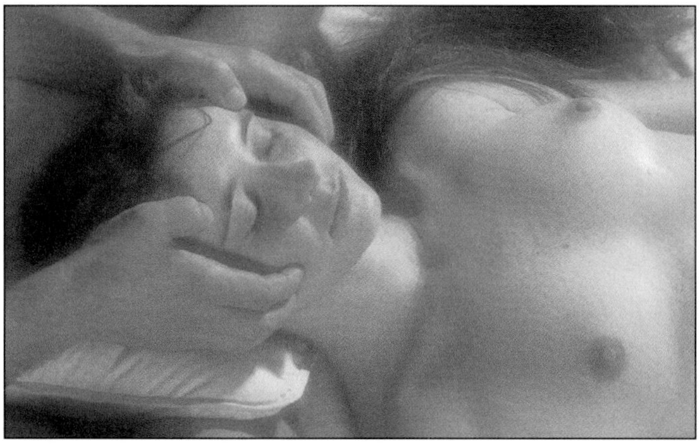

7 *Relaxing the cheeks helps the whole face to soften. Gently massage into the cheeks by moving your fingertips outwards in circular motions, then massage around the jaw, particularly at the joint.*

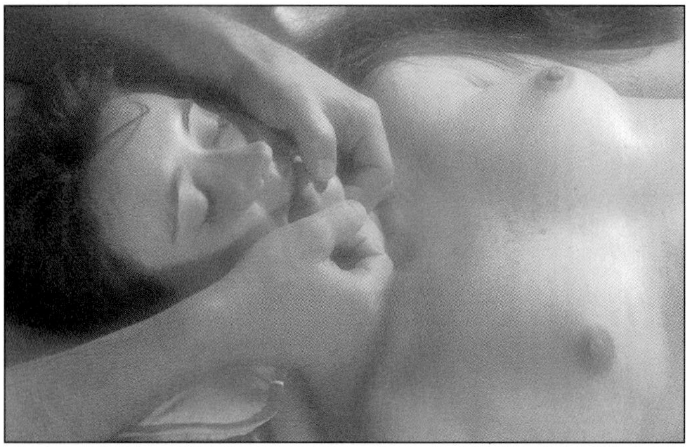

8 *Knead over your partner's chin with short, downward sliding thumb strokes, letting one thumb follow the other. Repeat these strokes up over both sides of her jawline.*

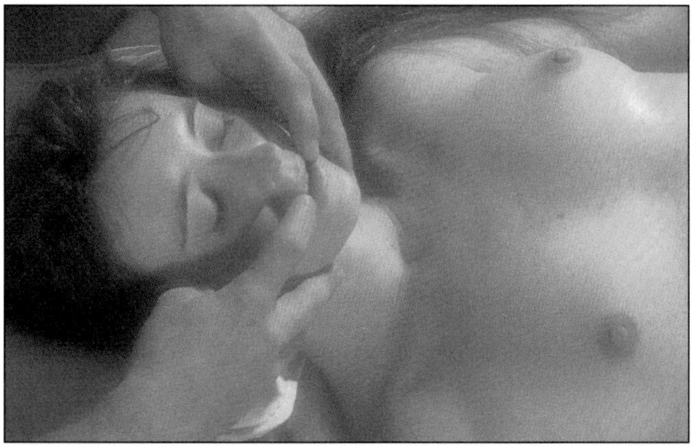

9 *Stroke intimately and softly with your fingertips around your partner's mouth and over her lips, lightly emphasizing their sensual contours.*

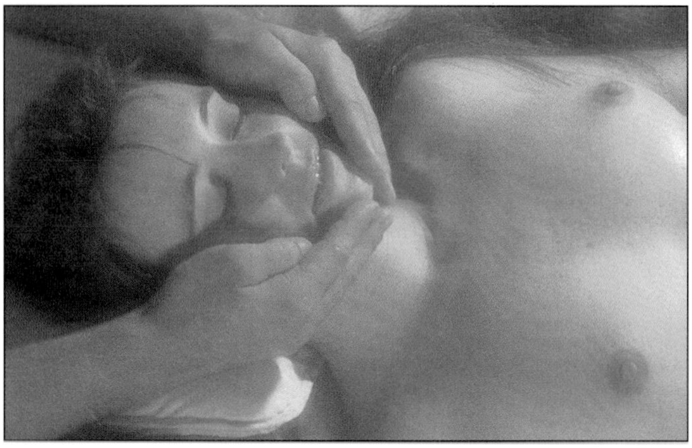

10 *Gently caress her throat by tenderly stroking up over the skin with your fingertips. Continue these soft strokes along the jawline with upward and outward sweeps of your hands and fingertips.*

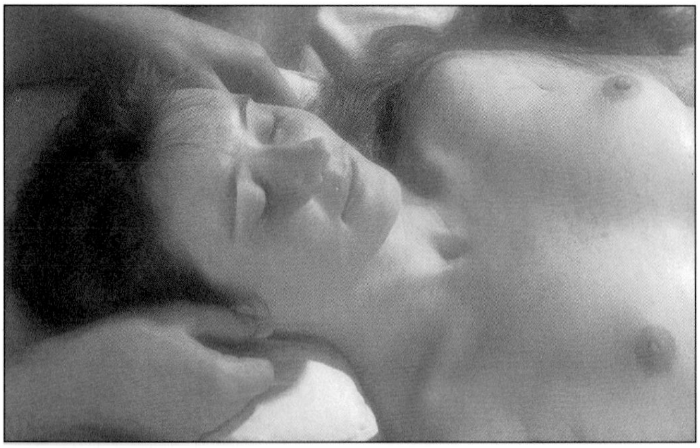

11 *Massage your partner's ears using your thumbs and fingertips to make small circular motions over the earlobes and around the ears. Lightly stroke over the back of the ears and around the inner surface.*

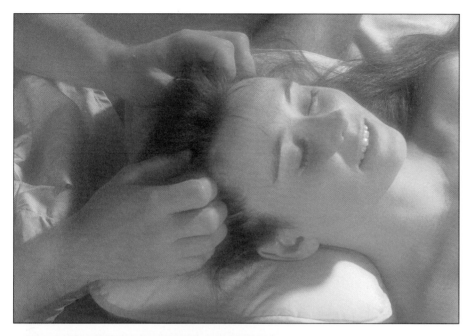

*12* A loving way to complete a face massage is to stroke your fingers gently through your partner's hair, taking away any remnants of tension from her head.

One of the best rewards for giving this massage is to see your partner's face soften and relax under the comfort and warmth of your hands. A good face massage induces feelings of peace and reassurance.

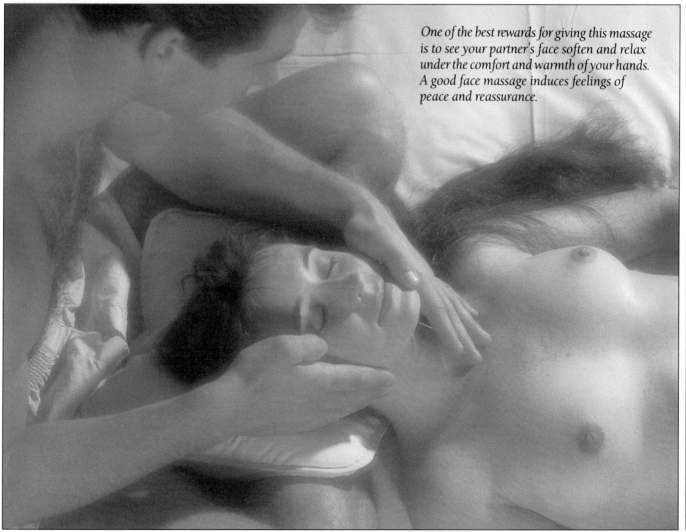

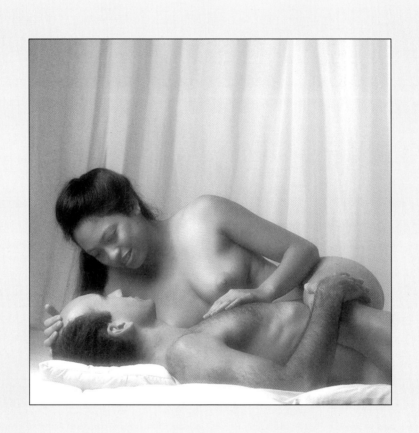

# Celebrating
# your sensuality

SENSUALITY ENCOMPASSES the whole body so
that every cell can become responsive and alive
to the joy of touch. In a truly sensual massage, while
your hands guide your strokes, your entire body
will become involved in sensuous play.
The combination of relaxation, stimulation,
teasing and laughter that results from a sensual
massage will heighten your responses
to each other as well as deepen
the intimacy between you.
In this programme, the massage focuses first
on your partner's back and then moves on
to the front with a series of strokes over the chest
and belly. It relaxes and tantalizes with soothing
and invigorating movements, and provides
you with the scope to be as playful
and adventurous as your mood allows. By
the time your partner turns over, both of
you will be ready to indulge in a total
celebration of sensual delight.

# Soothing strokes...

THE BACK OF THE BODY is always an excellent place to begin a sensual massage. If either of you feels at all inhibited or tense, it is the least threatening place to start, and its large surface will give you both time to relax together. It is an area that frequently receives little attention, yet the whole body can benefit enormously from the back being touched and soothed. A caring massage over this part of the body is one of the most effective ways of removing tension, relaxing the mind and generally raising your partner's spirits.

Sit or kneel by the side of your partner's back and start the massage by smoothing oil over the back and legs with large flowing strokes. Then you can begin to relax the back with the soft, sensual movements shown opposite.

*1 Bring your entire body into your movements as you stroke oil into your partner's back. Explore the whole of his back as you do so, letting your touch show your delight in his skin, his muscles – the feel of his whole body.*

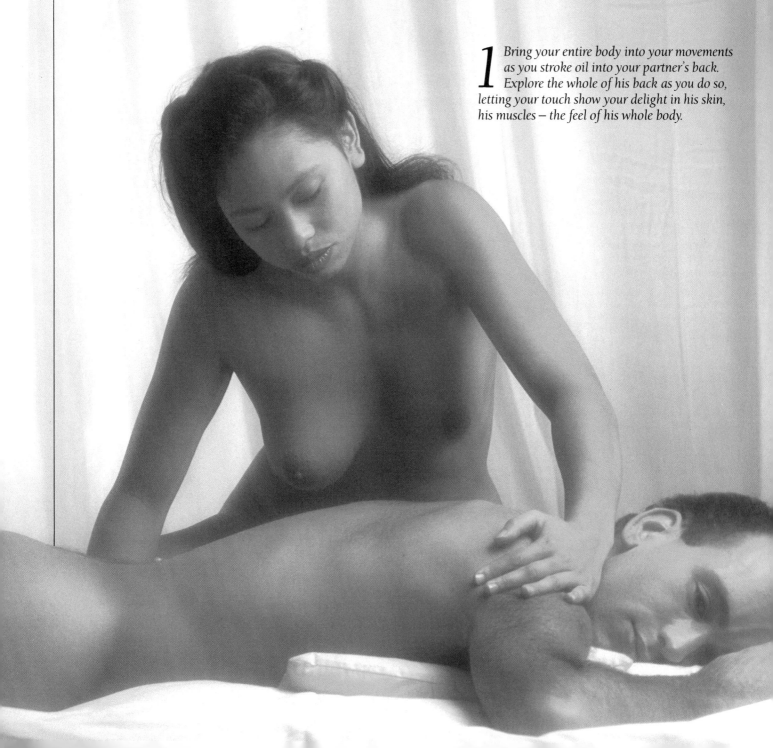

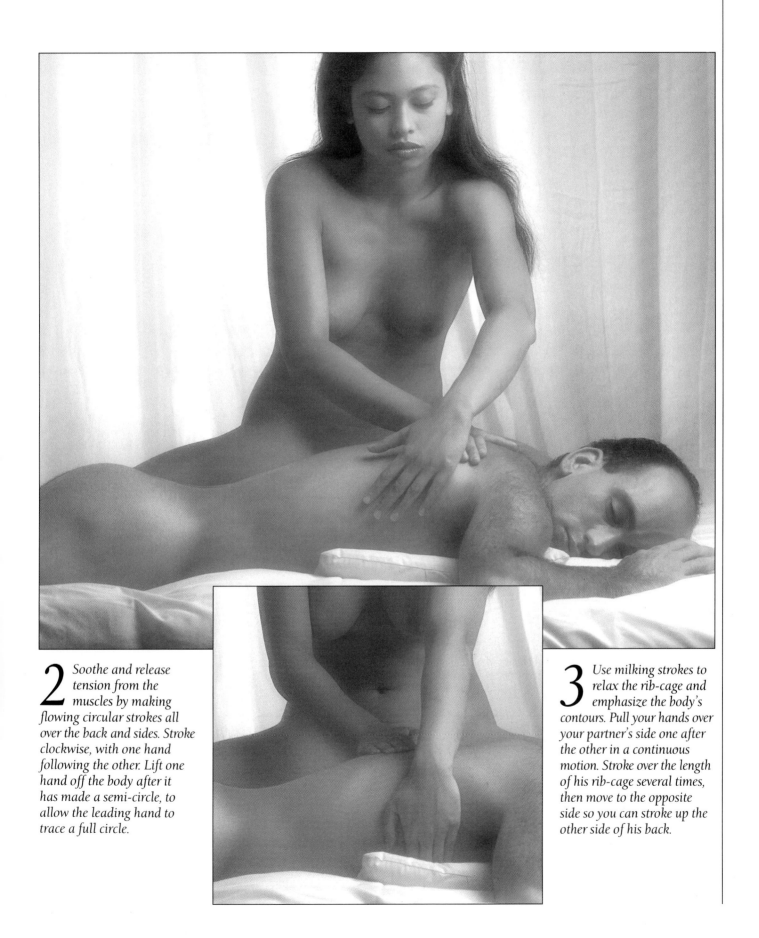

**2** *Soothe and release tension from the muscles by making flowing circular strokes all over the back and sides. Stroke clockwise, with one hand following the other. Lift one hand off the body after it has made a semi-circle, to allow the leading hand to trace a full circle.*

**3** *Use milking strokes to relax the rib-cage and emphasize the body's contours. Pull your hands over your partner's side one after the other in a continuous motion. Stroke over the length of his rib-cage several times, then move to the opposite side so you can stroke up the other side of his back.*

# Increasing the intimacy...

FOR CLOSER CONTACT and heightened sensuality, straddle your partner so he feels the warmth of your inner thighs as you massage him. Continue to relax his back with a series of sweeping strokes starting over his buttocks. Involve your whole body in these movements, and repeat them several times until you feel the muscles relaxing and melting under your touch.

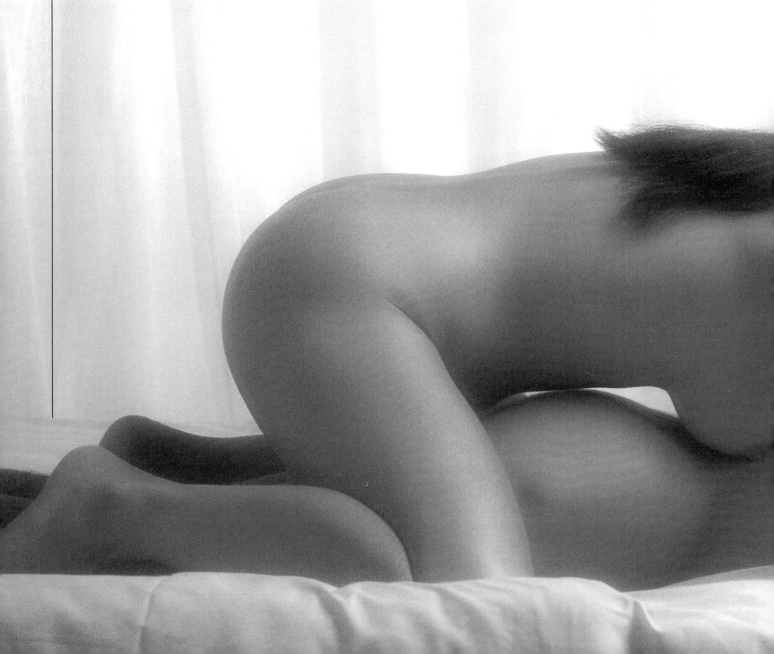

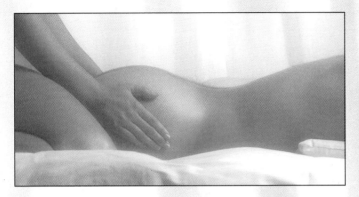

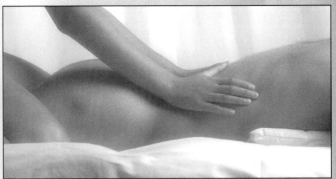

1 *Glide your hands from the base of the spine over the pelvis and hips, turning your wrists so your hands mould over the rounded form of your partner's buttocks. Sweep your hands in decreasing circular motions, following the contours of the buttocks, and then widen the movement to the original stroke.*

2 *Lean forwards as your hands progress up his back with the soothing movements of relaxing fan strokes. Support your weight with your knees and leg muscles to avoid causing any discomfort to your partner.*

3 *As your hands stroke over and around your partner's shoulders and upper arms, lower your body so your breasts gently brush against his back.*

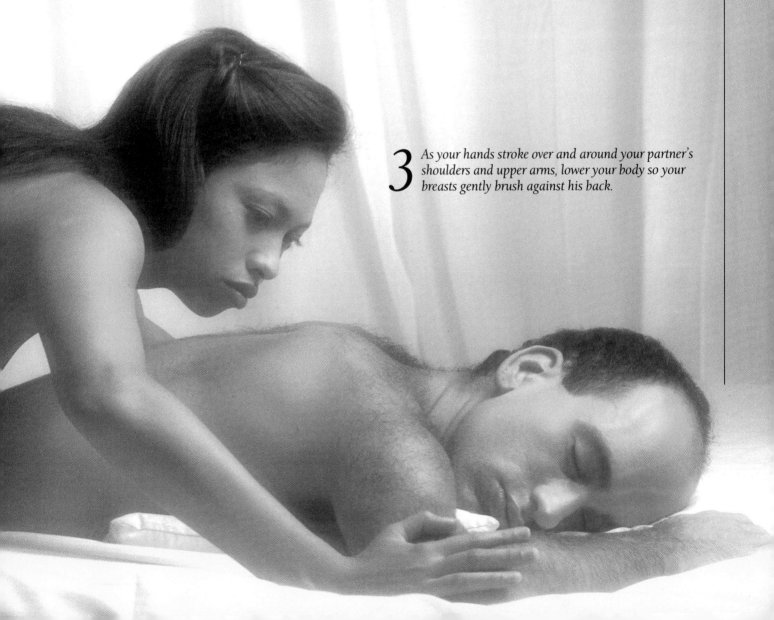

# Tantalizing play...

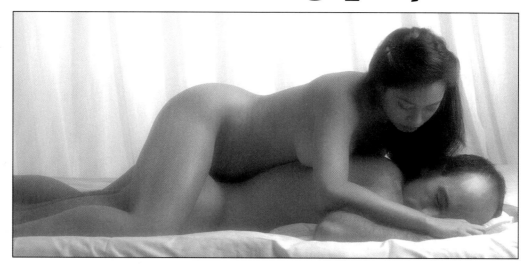

1 Lean fully over your partner's body. Tighten your thighs against the sides of his buttocks and slowly and sensually move your pelvis while you slide your body from side to side over the oiled surface of his skin. Let your belly and breasts rub softly against him.

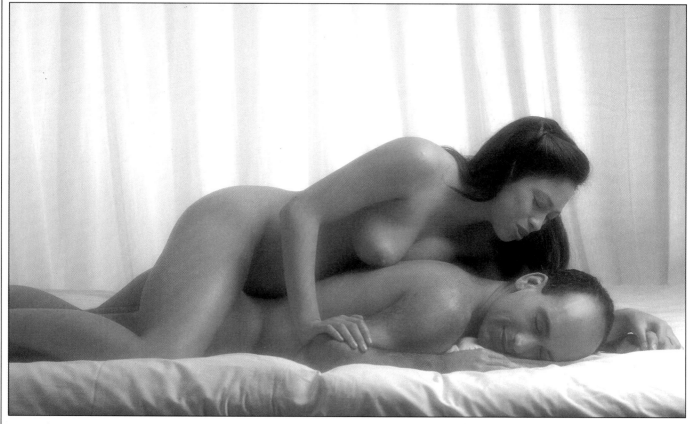

2 Tantalize and heighten your partner's senses by blowing softly onto his ear and the back of his neck. If you have long hair, excite him further by sweeping it lightly over his back. Keep your weight off your partner by supporting yourself on your knees and elbows.

3 Return to a kneeling position (see opposite), and rake your fingertips playfully down his back, running them from his shoulders down to his buttocks, to increase the vitality and vibrancy of his skin.

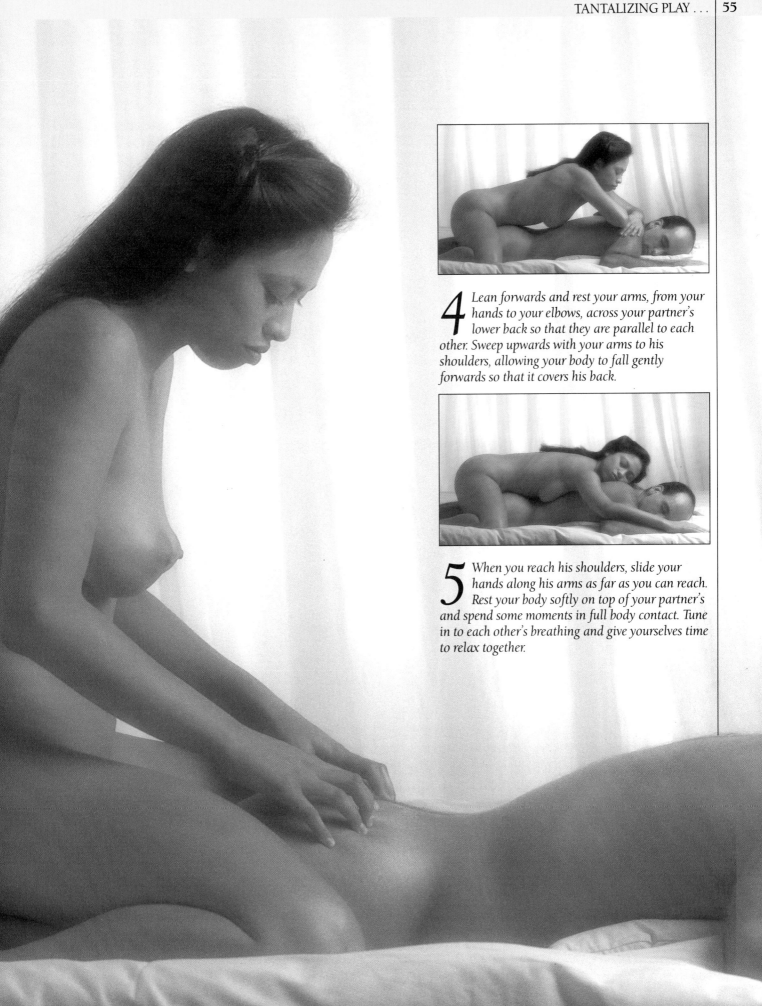

**4** Lean forwards and rest your arms, from your hands to your elbows, across your partner's lower back so that they are parallel to each other. Sweep upwards with your arms to his shoulders, allowing your body to fall gently forwards so that it covers his back.

**5** When you reach his shoulders, slide your hands along his arms as far as you can reach. Rest your body softly on top of your partner's and spend some moments in full body contact. Tune in to each other's breathing and give yourselves time to relax together.

# Lingering touches...

Wⁿᴴᴱⁿ ʸᴼᵁ FEEL READY, gently move off your partner's body and kneel between his knees so you can reach his buttocks and legs comfortably. Massage a little more oil into his legs if you need to, stroking downwards in the direction of the hair growth.

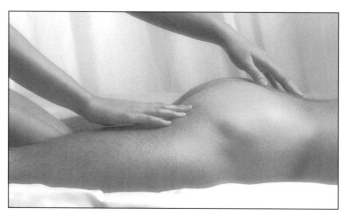

*1 Lightly stroke your fingers down your partner's lower back, over his buttocks and onto his thighs. Vary your pressure from soft to the barest of touches as you repeat these feather strokes. Then increase the pressure in your fingers and invigorate the area by covering it with raking strokes.*

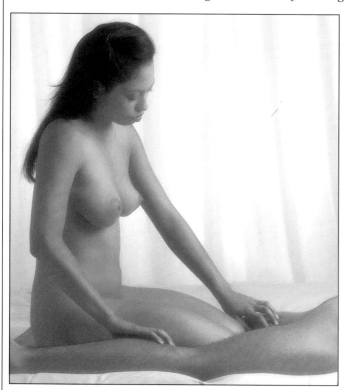

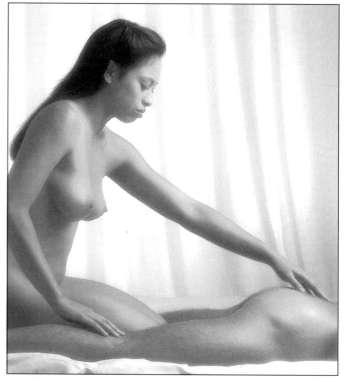

*2 Extend these raking strokes down your partner's inner thighs. Play with the speed and pressure of your strokes to increase the sensitivity of this area. Lighten your touch as you stroke over the back of the knees.*

*3 Teasingly feather stroke along your partner's legs, moving one hand after the other. Let your fingers slip softly onto and along his inner thighs as you stroke, and linger over the sensitive soft skin at the back of his knees.*

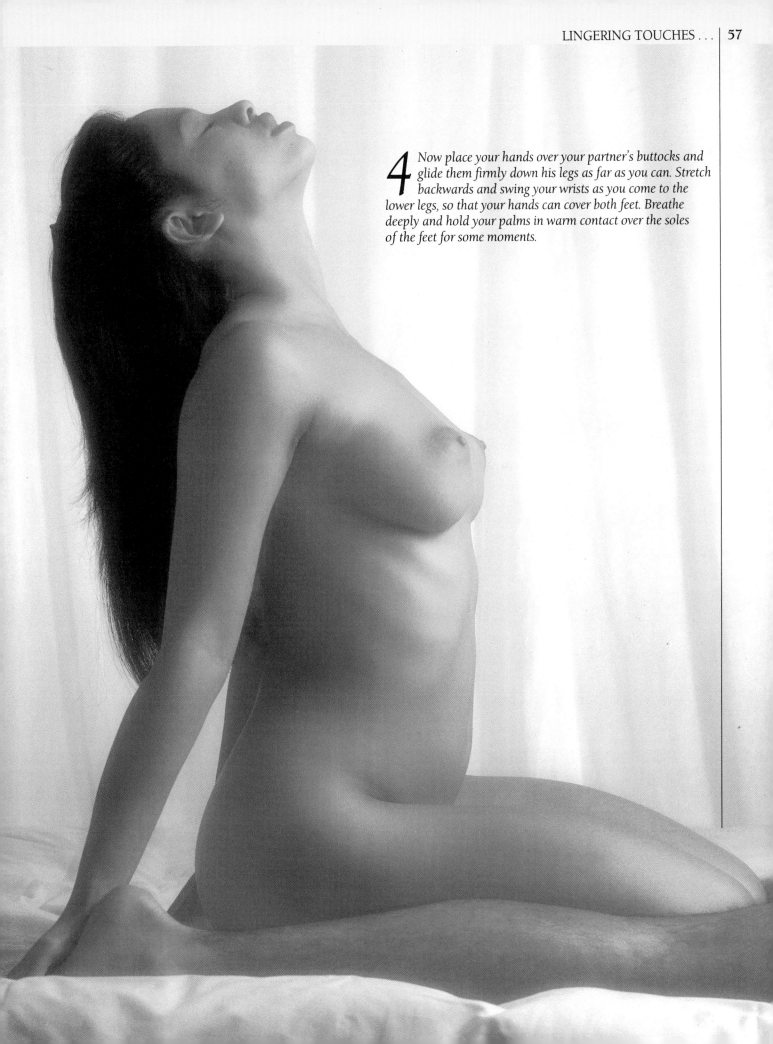

*4* Now place your hands over your partner's buttocks and glide them firmly down his legs as far as you can. Stretch backwards and swing your wrists as you come to the lower legs, so that your hands can cover both feet. Breathe deeply and hold your palms in warm contact over the soles of the feet for some moments.

# Heightening arousal ...

THE BUTTOCKS ARE a highly erotic area of the body and can hold
a lot of sexual feelings and tensions within their large, strong
muscles. Men, in particular, often feel sexually aroused by having
their buttocks massaged. Whereas until now your strokes have
mainly been soft and sensual, you can vary their tempo over the
buttocks to give a deep, thorough and invigorating
massage. Begin with several sweeping fan strokes to
cover the full surface of the buttocks, using your
hands and even the surface of your forearms. Then
massage all around the hips with the heels of your
hands. Increase and decrease the pressure and
speed of your strokes to create a stimulating
rhythm. Harmonize the deeper strokes
shown here from time to time by
sweeping your full hands over the
buttocks and pelvis and teasing
with feather-light finger strokes.

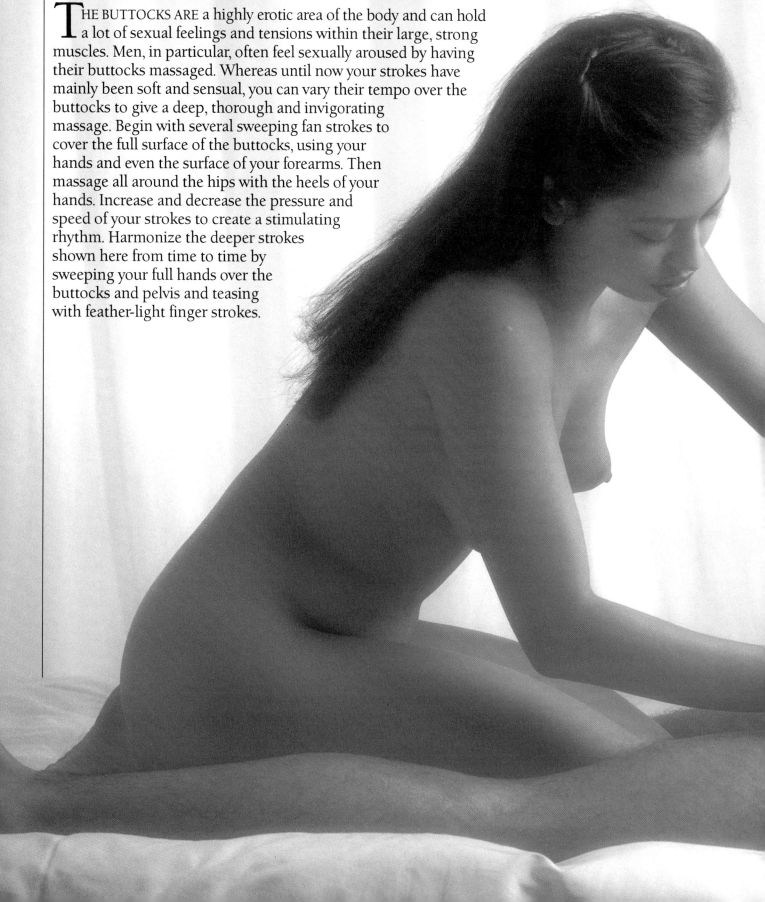

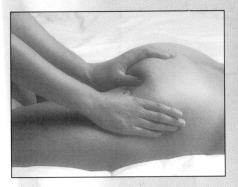

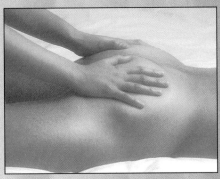

*2* Massage under and into the slopes where the buttocks and thighs meet by pressing your thumb pads into the crease of flesh and around the bones, making short, sliding strokes. Repeat these strokes several times.

*3* Place your hands over the fleshy cheeks of the buttocks and shake them lightly and rhythmically for an invigorating movement.

*1* Knead thoroughly over the fleshy area of the buttocks, lifting and rolling the flesh under your hands, pushing it between the fingers and thumbs in a wave-like motion.

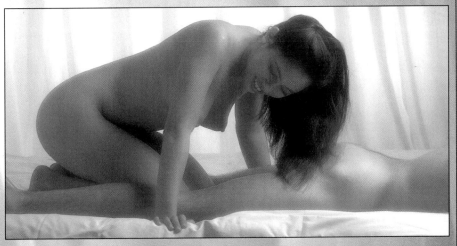

*4* Extend the teasing, playful nature of the last movement by sweeping your hair over your partner's buttocks and thighs. Arouse him further by letting him feel the soft caress of your breasts against his skin.

# Diffusing the feelings...

ONCE YOU ARE BOTH feeling aroused from the massage over the back of the body, heighten the sensuality by diffusing the feelings of sexuality so that they spread all over the body, making it totally alive and responsive. Do this by using your hands and body to extend this exquisite massage onto the front of your partner's body.

Playfully help your partner to roll over onto his ·back so that you can massage his belly and chest. The belly is a vulnerable, unprotected area. By helping it to relax through massage, you can assist your partner to deeper and fuller breathing, which leads in turn to greater vitality and heightened emotional and sexual responses.

*1 Sit or kneel by your partner's waist and spread a little oil firmly but gently over his belly, hips, and chest, and the sides of his body. Let your own body move gracefully with your strokes.*

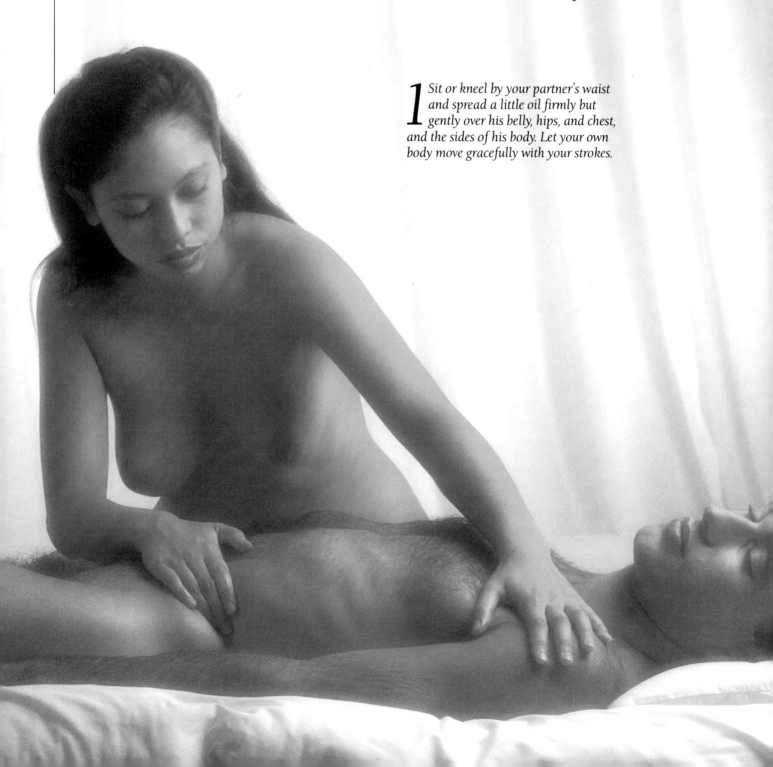

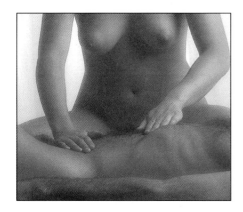

**2** Place one hand just below the rib-cage and the other below the navel. Wait some moments until you feel the belly relaxing beneath your hands, then begin to slide them over the abdomen, making large circular strokes in a clockwise direction.

(Right) Decrease these circles gradually into the centre of the belly and then expand them outwards again. Slowly deepen the pressure of your strokes.

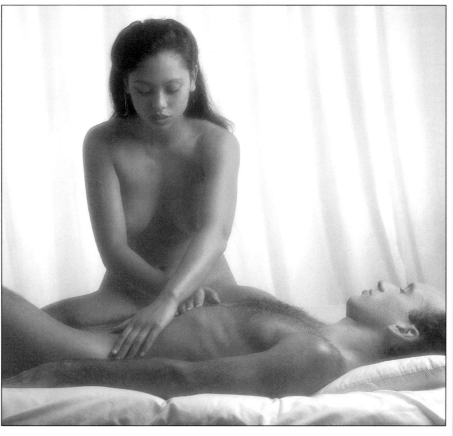

**3** Loosen the sides of the abdomen with milking strokes running from the hips to the rib-cage and back again. Slide your fingers from under the back of the body right over the sides as your hands pull towards the centre of the belly. Work the strokes up and down several times and then repeat them from the other side of your partner's body.

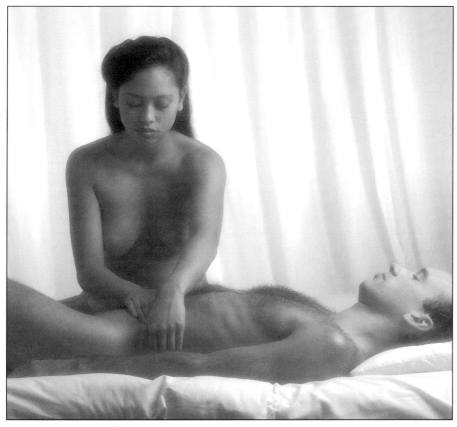

# Intensifying the pleasure...

THIS SERIES OF STROKES will help your partner to breathe more deeply into his chest. In doing this, it can also release his more subtle emotions, leaving him free to surrender himself to the pleasures of your massage. These strokes form a continuous, flowing movement that covers the upper body. To heighten arousal, straddle your partner's hips lightly, just above his pubic bone, taking care not to press your weight down on his body. Apply a little oil to the body as you massage and repeat the movements several times, varying your pressure and speed from slow and soft to fast and strong, but always returning to soft, sensual strokes.

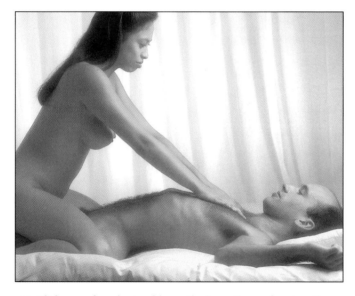

1 *Slide your hands steadily up the breastbone, fanning them out over the top of the chest to pass under the collar-bone towards the shoulders. Let yourself fall gently forwards as you lean your body-weight into this stroke to widen and stretch the upper chest muscles.*

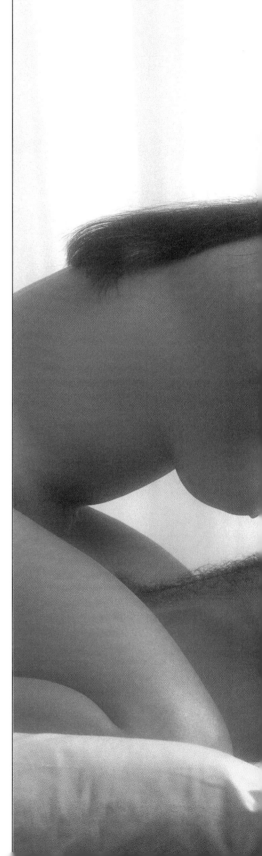

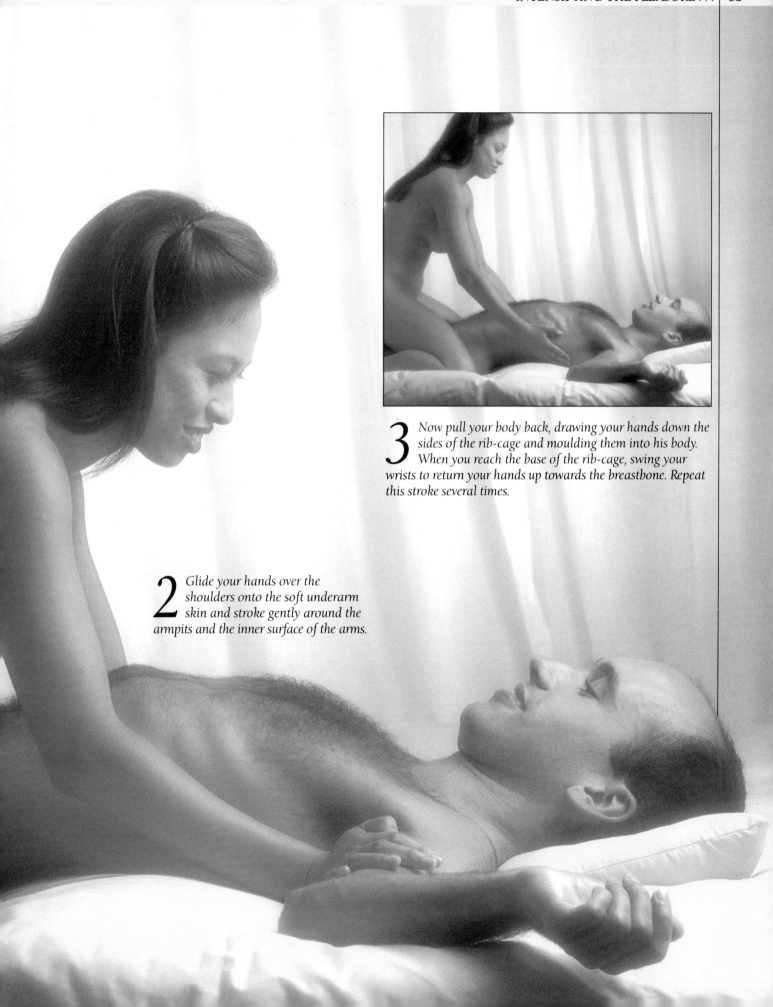

**3** *Now pull your body back, drawing your hands down the sides of the rib-cage and moulding them into his body. When you reach the base of the rib-cage, swing your wrists to return your hands up towards the breastbone. Repeat this stroke several times.*

**2** *Glide your hands over the shoulders onto the soft underarm skin and stroke gently around the armpits and the inner surface of the arms.*

# The full body caress...

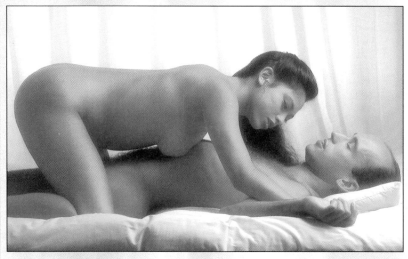

*1* *Delight yourself and your partner by slowly lowering your body over his, keeping your hands and knees on the mattress to support your weight. Turn your body smoothly and softly from side to side to caress him with tantalizing brushes of your breasts, belly and hair.*

2 Make a last sweeping stroke up your partner's body to end with an exciting and playful bondage hold. Raise your body and place your hands over the base of the breastbone. Sweep them upwards, over the upper chest and shoulders and onto the arms. Lean your weight gently into your hands as they rest on the arms. From this position, you can both relax into eye contact with each other, one of the strongest and yet most vulnerable ways to communicate your excitement and feelings for each other.

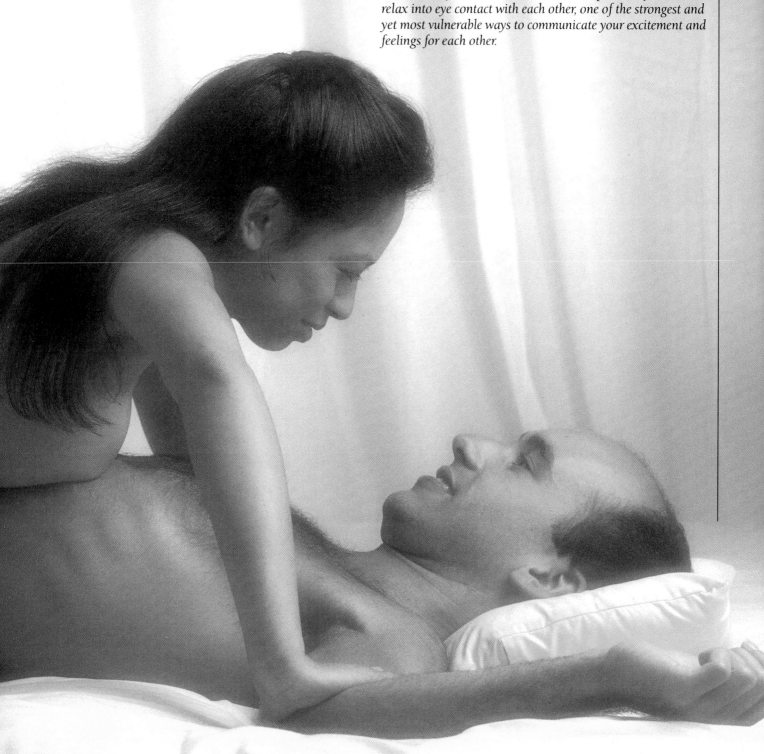

*Within a loving relationship,
sensuality opens the doors to pleasure
where your bodies become an endless playground
of discovery to be shared
with one another . . .*

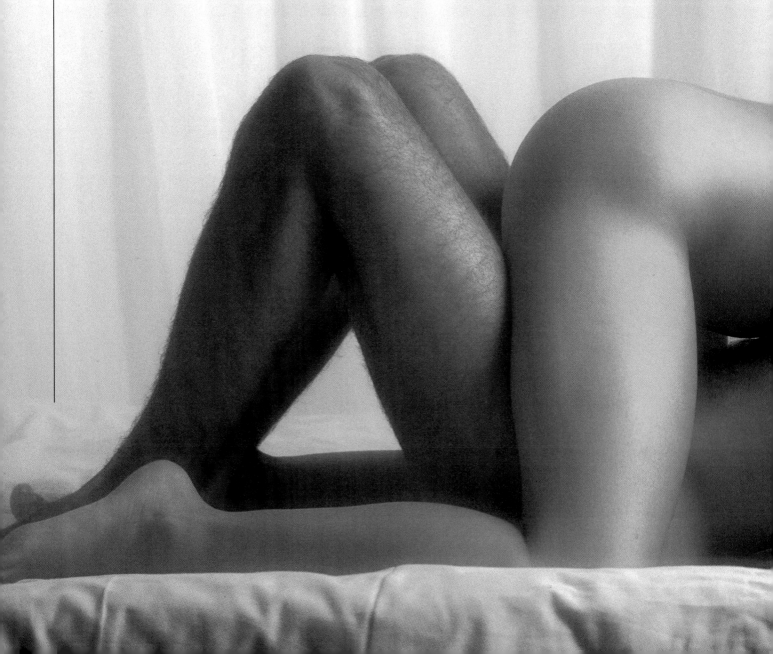

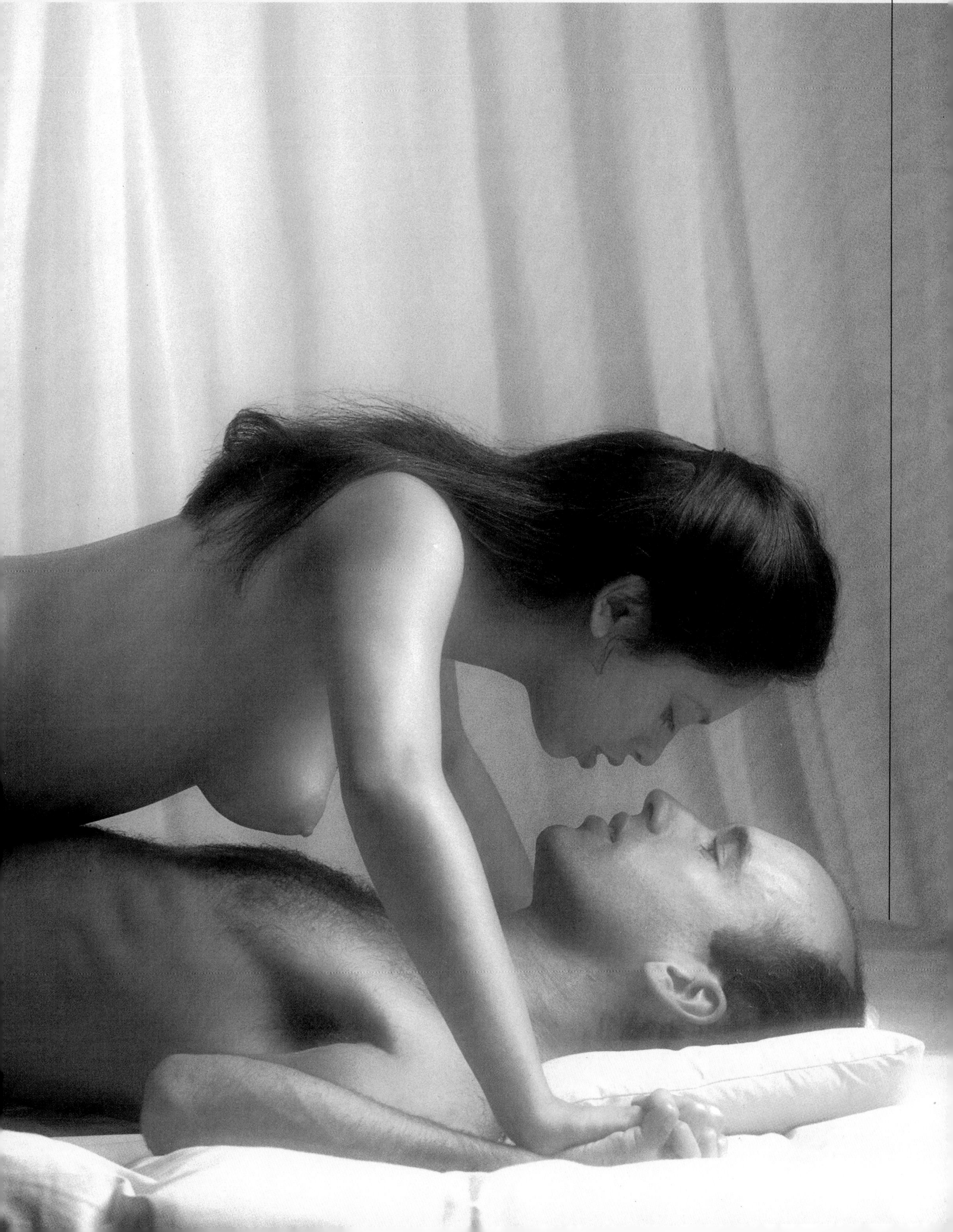

# Water play

WITH ITS UNIQUE QUALITIES, water makes an inspiring setting for intimate and sensual contact between you and your partner. For water not only cleanses, it refreshes, revitalizes, soothes and relaxes. Water makes you feel buoyant and playful, soft and sensual. Being in water, you are natural and naked. So share the time you spend bathing with your partner and make it an event in itself, or a prelude to an intimate massage . . .

A jacuzzi bath is a luxurious way to relax with your partner. While the jets of water massage and invigorate different parts of your body, the steamy heat of the water soothes your muscles. It is the perfect sensual experience for both of you to share.

**Water caresses** (right)
*Let the water soothe and revitalize you as you caress each other's body, and enjoy the intimacy that this brings.*

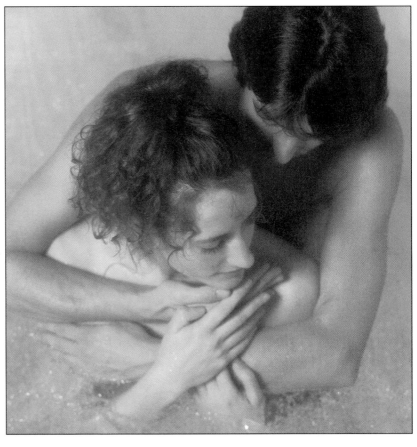

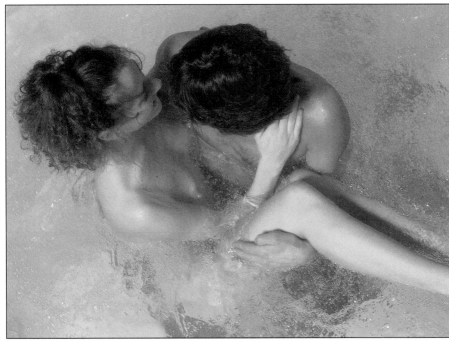

**Whirlpool baths**
*The swirling water, bubbling currents and steamy atmosphere of a jacuzzi ensure a highly pleasurable experience. Relax together and relish the opportunity that such time brings to touch, massage and play together in the water.*

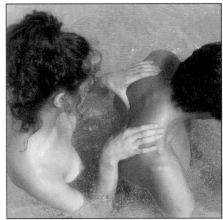

**Water massage**
*Make the most of the soothing effects of the warm, flowing water by massaging along your partner's spine and into his shoulders and neck. A water massage will be a truly relaxing occasion.*

**Playing with water** (opposite)
*Luxuriate in the sensations of the water as it flows over your skin, caressing and soothing your muscles. Trickle it through your fingers over your partner's body.*

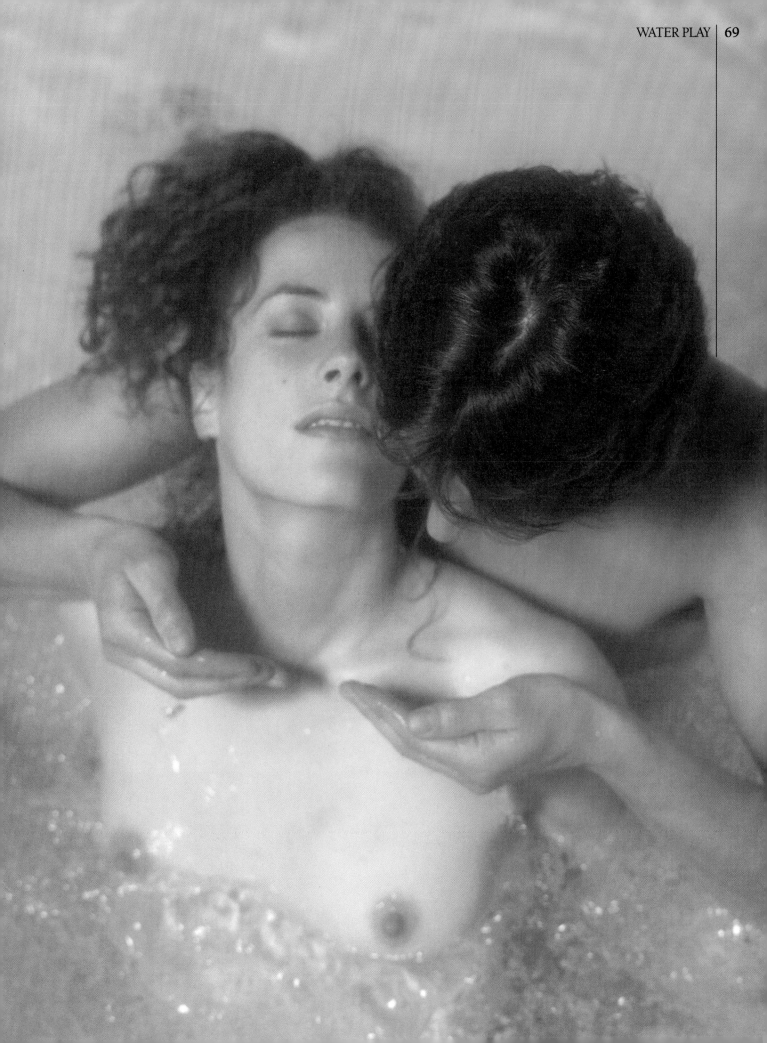

# Sensual bathing

$S$OAKING TOGETHER IN A BATH TUB, you can turn what may seem mundane, cleansing tasks into a ritual of delightful intimacy. Soaping your partner can be an excuse for giving a soapy, sensual massage, the slippery lather helping your hands to slide over and around your partner's body contours. By using massage strokes as you caringly shampoo each other's hair, you can transform a hair wash into a delightful experience. After your bath, continue this luxurious pampering play by taking time to dry each other with warm towels and massaging body lotion into each other's skin.

**Exploring each other**
*Every moment of shared bathing can be made special. While you spend time soaping each other, use the rich creamy lather as a lotion to help your hands slide over, explore and relax your partner's body.*

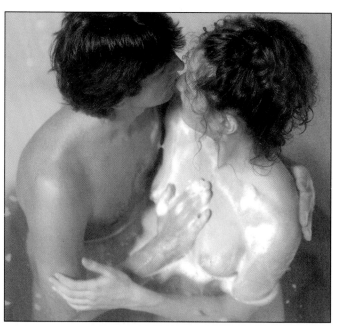

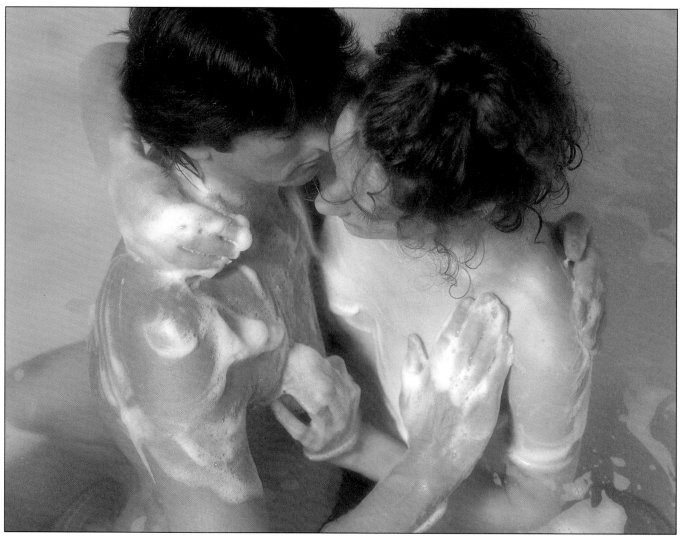

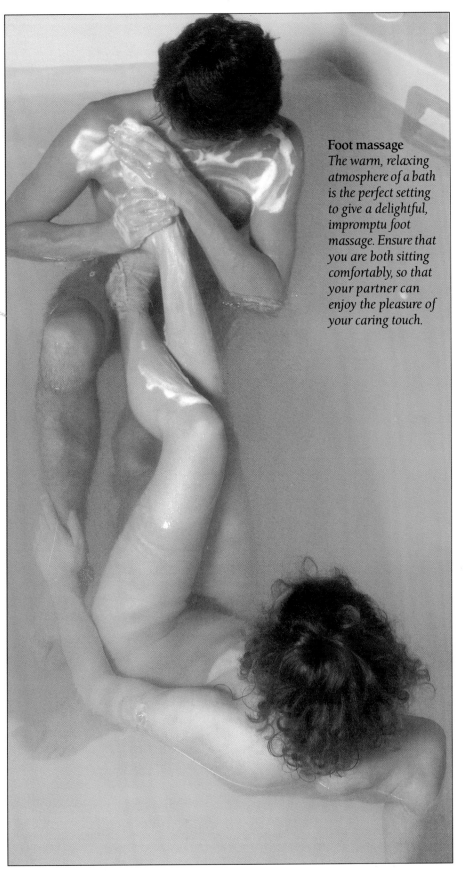

**Foot massage**
*The warm, relaxing atmosphere of a bath is the perfect setting to give a delightful, impromptu foot massage. Ensure that you are both sitting comfortably, so that your partner can enjoy the pleasure of your caring touch.*

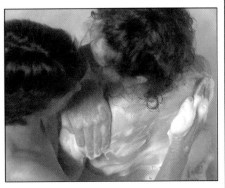

**Back massage**
*Tired, tense muscles melt easily under your loving hands during a bath-time massage. Take advantage of the naturally relaxing and healing effects of water and of its warmth on the body's muscles by giving your partner a soothing shoulder, neck and back massage.*

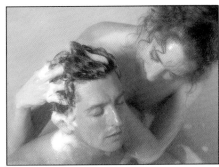

**Shampooing**
*One of the most pleasurable bath-time experiences you can have is to relax your whole body in warm, steaming water while your partner transforms a hair shampoo into a caring head massage.*

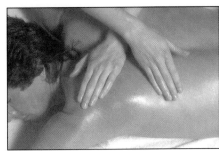

**After bathing**
*Increase the physical closeness and intimacy between you after bathing together by applying an enriching skin lotion. Gently massage into the muscles as the lotion soaks into the skin.*

# Showering together

TAKING A SHOWER TOGETHER provides the ideal opportunity for fun and sensuality. The closeness of your bodies, your movements together, and the gentle force of the water running down your skin can turn a simple shower into a spontaneously erotic occasion. Water has the ability to wash away tensions and lighten your spirits as it rains down on you.

After initially relaxing yourselves under the stream of water, soap each other all over, letting your hands explore each other's body. Slide against the soapy surfaces of each other's skin in a slippery full body massage.

For a totally refreshing experience that will invigorate the skin and stimulate the blood circulation, leaving you feeling tinglingly alive, lightly massage your partner with a loofah. At the end of the shower, towel each other dry with soft, warm towels. A brisk rub down stimulates and warms the body; caressing the skin and enfolding your partner in towels has a soothing effect.

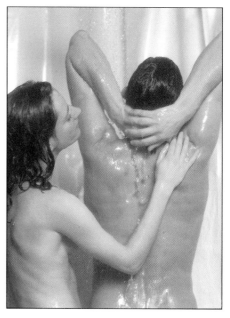

**Flowing water** (*above and below*)
*Water running against the skin produces an almost alchemical effect on the mind and the body. It revitalizes and refreshes, awakening the spirit and transforming and lightening your mood.*

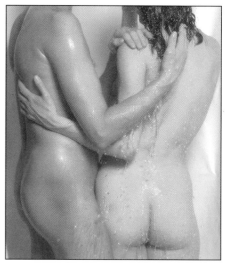

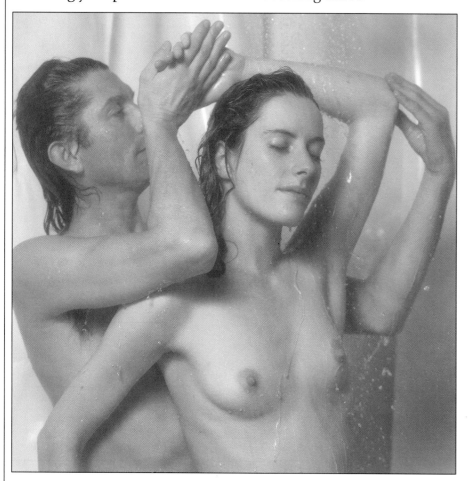

**Showering**
*Refresh yourselves and enhance your physical relationship by showering together. Morning or night, or any time of day, let this become a ritual to express your sensuality and bring you closer together. Enjoy the opportunity for full naked contact in the exhilarating and natural setting of a shower.*

**Water on the skin** (*opposite*)
*When you shower with your partner, let the healing effects of the water benefit you both. Delight in the way it feels as it runs down your body, emphasizing the smooth texture of your skin.*

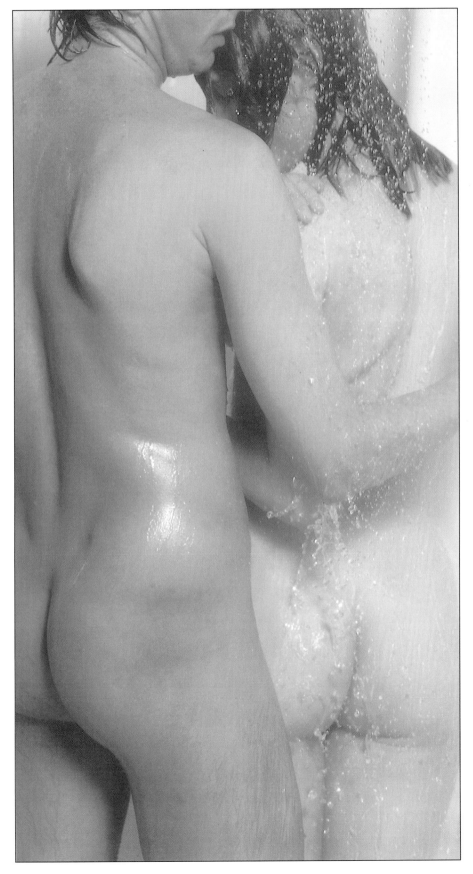

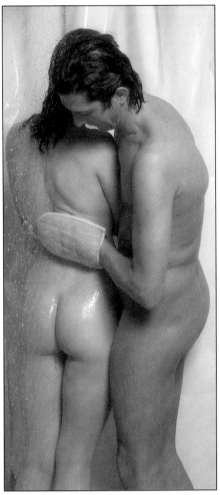

**Invigorating the skin** (*above*)
*Briskly rub all over your partner's body with a loofah, moving from the bottom to the top of the body. This will revitalize her skin, leaving her feeling energized and tingling all over.*

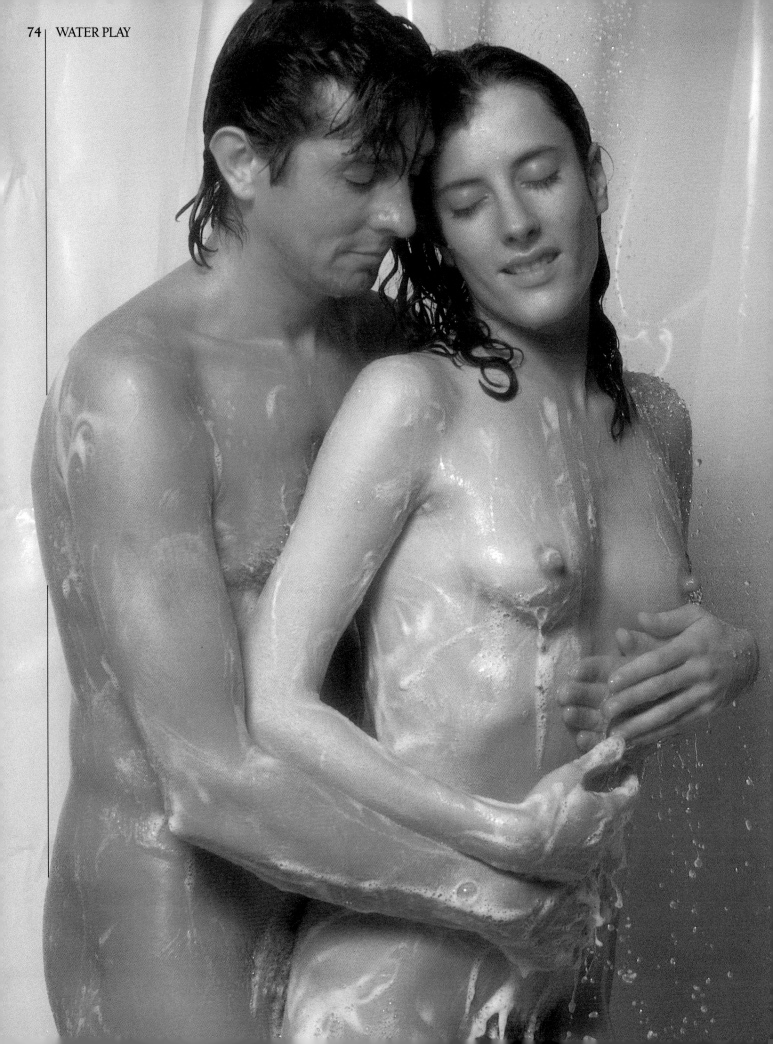

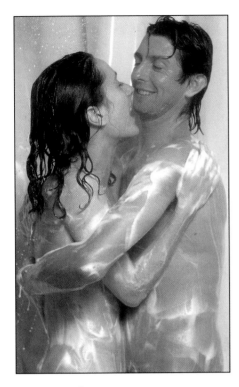

**Shower caressing** (*above and below*)
*Embrace beneath the stream of water and let it wash away the rivulets of soap bubbles from your skin.*

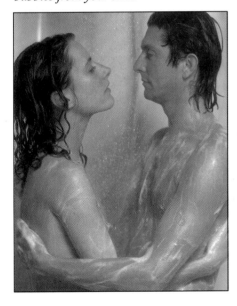

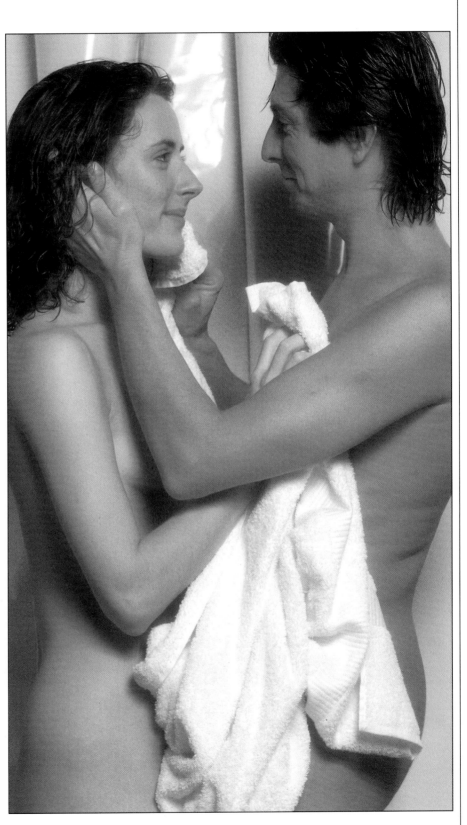

**Shower soaping** (*opposite*)
*Smooth the silky, soft, soapy lather into one another's skin. Come close together and try sliding your lathered bodies gently against each other.*

**Towel drying**
*Turn drying each other into a playful and caring experience. With warm, dry towels, tenderly wipe the wetness from each other's face, and gently pat each other's body dry. The simplest gesture can be a statement of love.*

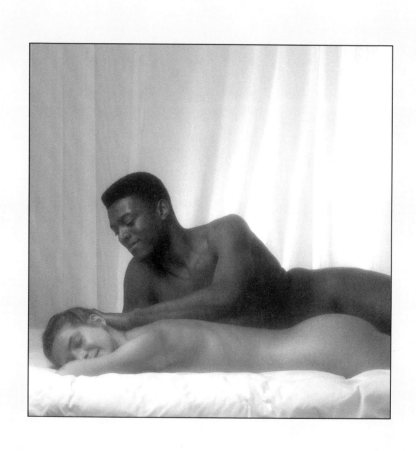

# Awakening the body

I N A BUSY WORLD, it is important to create time together to maintain the intimacy and closeness that nourish a relationship. Yet the stresses and strains of the day's events can often rob you of the emotional and physical resources you need to enjoy these precious moments together. On occasions when you are feeling energetic and communicative while your partner is tired, share your resources in a way that will benefit you both by giving your partner a caring and restorative sensual massage.

The following massage sequence is aimed at relaxing and revitalizing your partner, and gives you the opportunity to communicate your concern and tenderness through touch. Designed to be a tonic for the whole body, its upward strokes help to stimulate the circulation, which restores energy, while the combination of soothing and invigorating strokes will relax tense, tight muscles, leaving your partner feeling refreshed, stimulated and responsive.

# Releasing & reviving...

A FOOT MASSAGE helps the whole body to relax
while also stimulating the nervous system
through the thousands of nerve endings that lie in
the soles of the feet. It is both physically and
psychologically soothing, and leaves the body
feeling totally refreshed. Stroke a little oil down the
legs before you start. Any oil remaining on your
hands will be sufficient for the feet. Too much
oil can prevent you from getting a firm grip and
will make your strokes feel ticklish.
Massage one foot at a time.

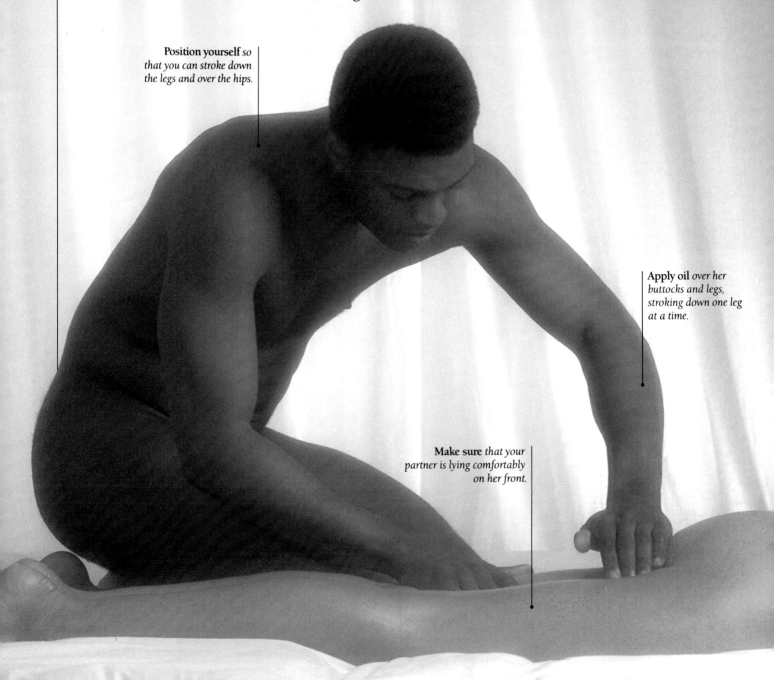

**Position yourself** *so
that you can stroke down
the legs and over the hips.*

**Apply oil** *over her
buttocks and legs,
stroking down one leg
at a time.*

**Make sure** *that your
partner is lying comfortably
on her front.*

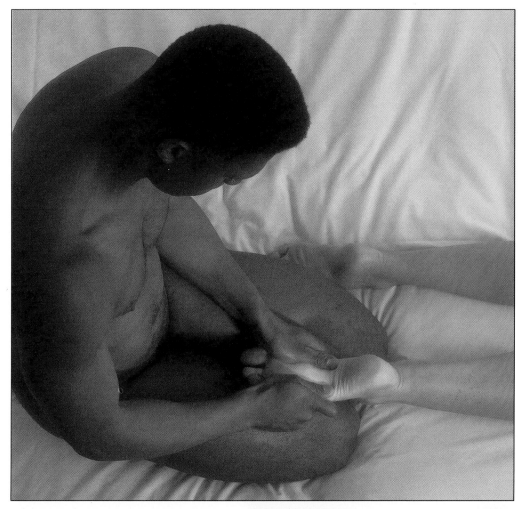

*1 Lift and support your partner's foot with both hands, placing your fingers firmly under the instep. Create a good stretch by sliding your heels and thumbs steadily from the centre of the sole outwards to the edge of the foot. Repeat this stroke to cover the surface of the sole.*

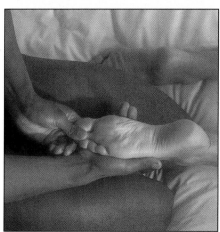

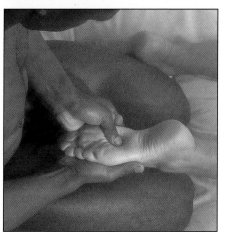

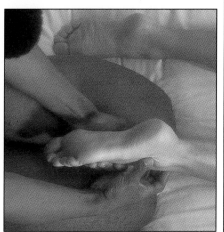

*2 Hold the foot with one hand and use your other hand to make the following strokes. With your thumb and forefinger, pull gently but firmly from the base to the tip of each toe, starting with the little toe. Pass the foot from one hand to the other whenever necessary.*

*3 Massage consistently over the whole surface of the sole, making tiny rotations with your thumb tips. Deepen the pressure as you feel the muscles under the skin relaxing. These strokes stimulate countless nerve endings in the foot, revitalizing the entire body.*

*4 Ankles take a lot of strain and benefit enormously from some gentle massage. Stroke around the ankle bones with your thumbs and fingertips. Relax the back of the ankle area by making small circular motions with the heels of your hands.*

# Stimulating strokes...

RELAX EACH LEG with the following series of firm, sweeping strokes, moulding your hands over the full length of the leg and the buttocks. Repeat these strokes several times so that they become one continuous movement. Once you feel that the leg has relaxed, invigorate the muscles in the calf and thigh with some deeper kneading strokes. Work on one leg first, then repeat the strokes on the other. To start, kneel by or over the feet in a position that allows you to stretch over your partner's body.

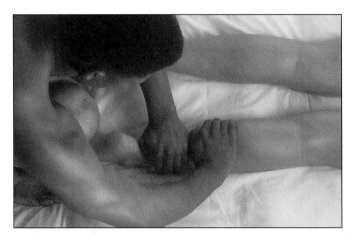

*1 Place your hands parallel to each other yet facing in opposite directions across the back of the ankle and the lower leg. Slide them upwards with a steady, even pressure, moulding them into the shape of the leg. Lessen your pressure as you pass over the sensitive area at the back of the knee, and continue the stroke over the thigh.*

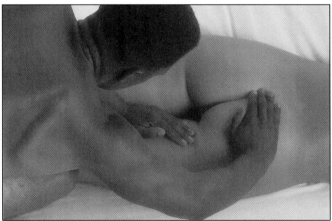

*Glide your upper hand smoothly over the buttock to encircle the pelvis and hip, while your lower hand slips onto and waits on the soft skin of the inner thigh. As you make this stroke, move your full hand steadily and lovingly as it slowly encompasses the contours of the body to emphasize its full sensuality.*

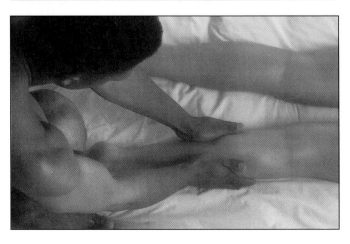

*When both hands are parallel on the thigh, pull them steadily down the sides of the leg towards the heel, drawing the stroke out of both sides of the foot. Repeat this whole sensual movement several times so that it feels like one flowing, continuous motion.*

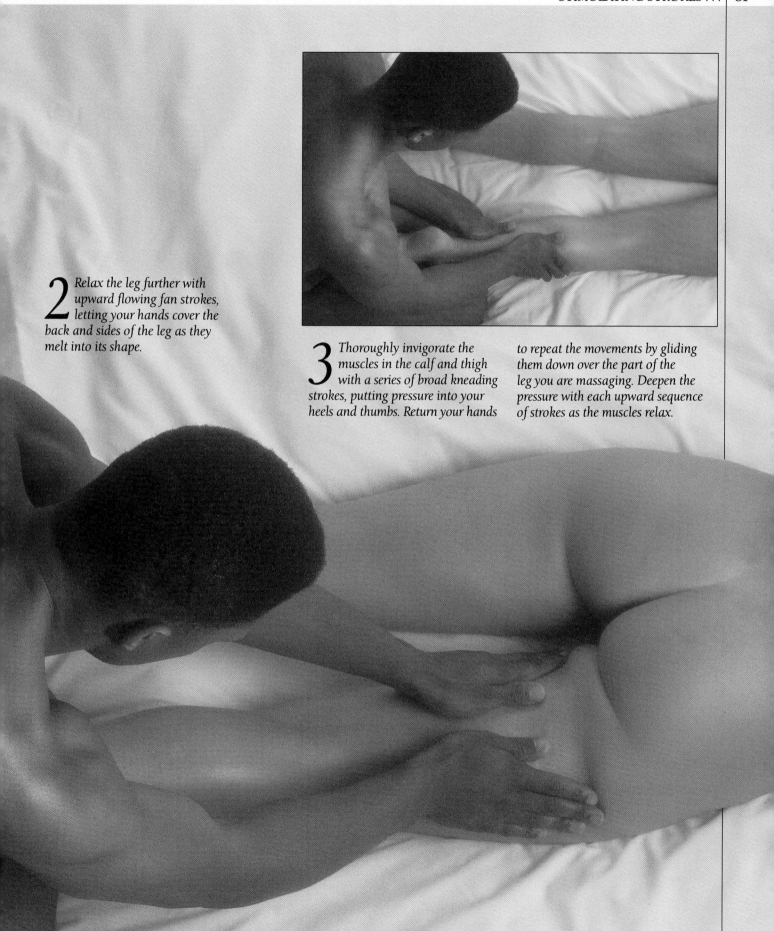

**2** Relax the leg further with upward flowing fan strokes, letting your hands cover the back and sides of the leg as they melt into its shape.

**3** Thoroughly invigorate the muscles in the calf and thigh with a series of broad kneading strokes, putting pressure into your heels and thumbs. Return your hands to repeat the movements by gliding them down over the part of the leg you are massaging. Deepen the pressure with each upward sequence of strokes as the muscles relax.

# Sensual contours...

AFTER YOU'VE MASSAGED both feet and legs, straddle your partner's thighs, or if you prefer, kneel at her side so you can sweep your hands easily over her buttocks and hips. If you are kneeling astride her, take care not to bring your weight down onto her. As you repeat the movements described below, gradually increase the pressure and speed of your strokes to bring heat and vitality to the area.

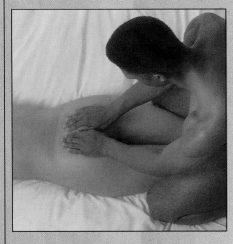
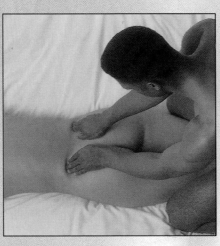
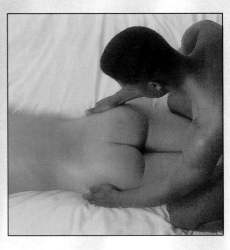

**1** Place both hands over the base of your partner's spine and move them steadily upwards and outwards in opposite directions.

Let your fingertips slide into and stretch the tissue just above the pelvic bone, to ease away any tension that may be stored in the lower back.

Continue the stroke around her hips and under her buttocks, moulding your hands into their full sensual contours. Return your hands lightly over the buttocks to the base of the spine, and repeat the stroke several times.

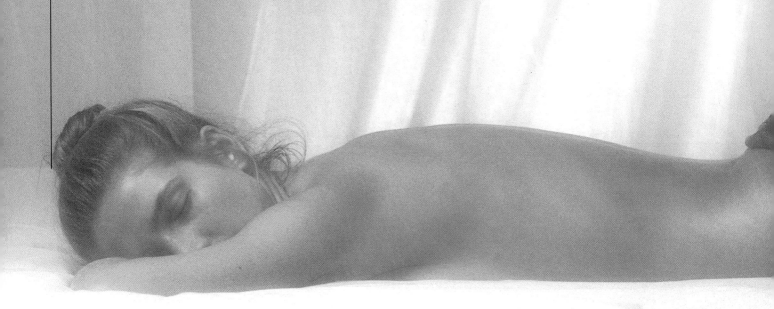

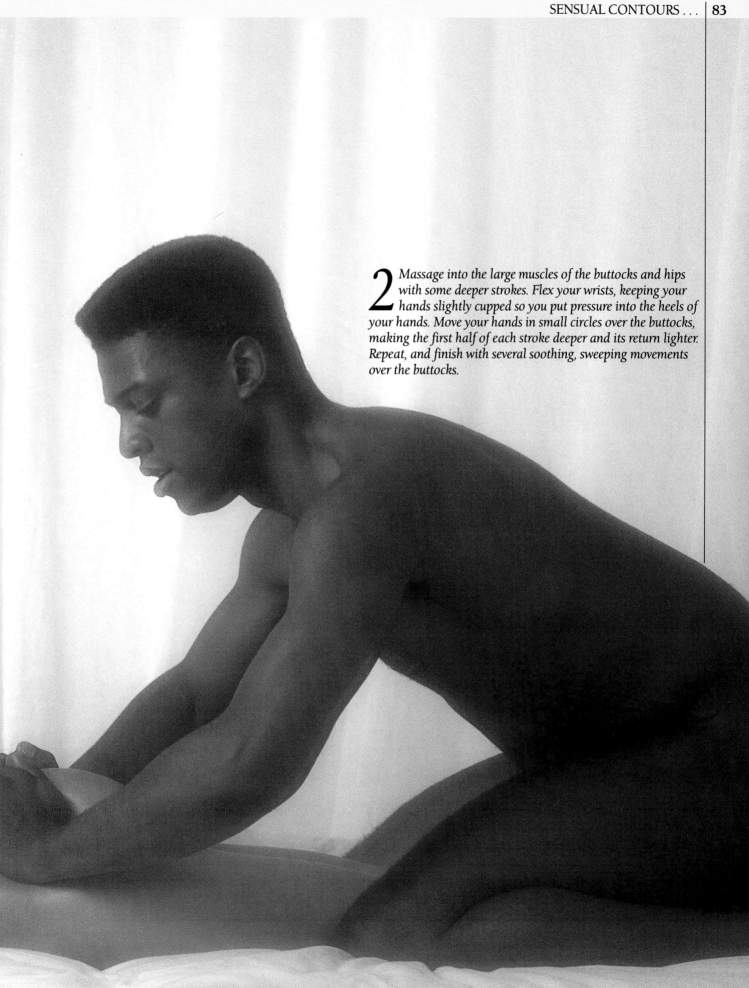

2 Massage into the large muscles of the buttocks and hips with some deeper strokes. Flex your wrists, keeping your hands slightly cupped so you put pressure into the heels of your hands. Move your hands in small circles over the buttocks, making the first half of each stroke deeper and its return lighter. Repeat, and finish with several soothing, sweeping movements over the buttocks.

# Soothing the back . . .

BEFORE YOU START to massage, smooth a little oil over the whole area. Soothe away the tension that so often gathers in the back, the neck and the shoulders with a series of sweeping fan strokes. Repeat these several times, letting your hands yield into the curves and softness of your partner's body until you feel the whole area loosening under your touch. Once you feel the muscles relax you can release them further with some more invigorating kneading. Blend these deeper strokes into the sensuality of your massage by sweeping your hands tenderly over your partner's back from time to time.

**APPLYING OIL TO THE BACK**

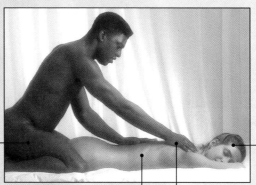

**Support your** *weight with your knees and your leg muscles.*

**Let your partner** *move her head from time to time.*

**Stroke a little** *oil into your partner's back and over her shoulders.*

**Cover the back** *with soft, flowing strokes as you anoint it.*

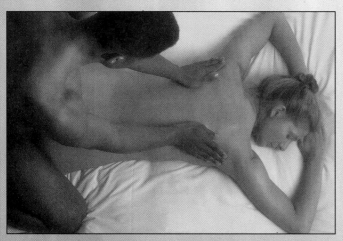

*1 Soothe the back with a series of fan strokes. Place your hands on each side of your partner's spine. Glide them upwards then fan them out over her back. Widen the movement to cover the sides of her rib-cage too. When your strokes reach the upper back, sweep your hands over the shoulders, then return them down the sides of the body.*

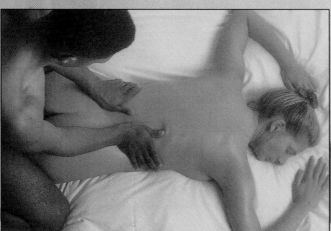

*2 Once you feel your partner relaxing, massage more vigorously up her back with broad kneading strokes, putting pressure into your heels and thumbs. Spend time on specific tension areas, such as the lower back.*

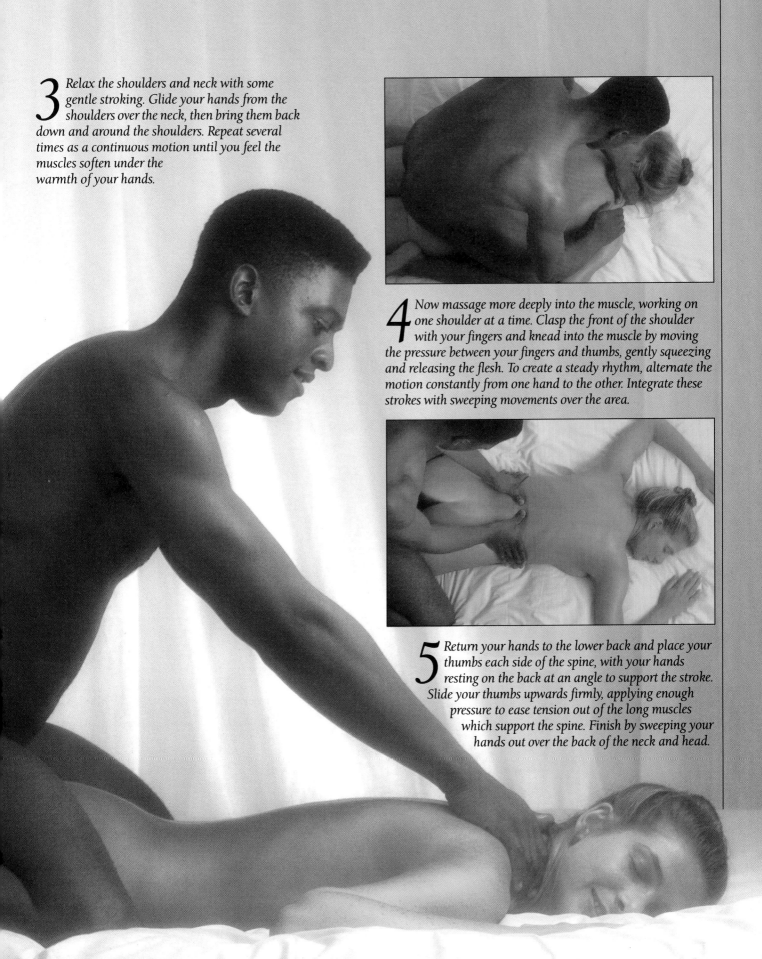

**3** *Relax the shoulders and neck with some gentle stroking. Glide your hands from the shoulders over the neck, then bring them back down and around the shoulders. Repeat several times as a continuous motion until you feel the muscles soften under the warmth of your hands.*

**4** *Now massage more deeply into the muscle, working on one shoulder at a time. Clasp the front of the shoulder with your fingers and knead into the muscle by moving the pressure between your fingers and thumbs, gently squeezing and releasing the flesh. To create a steady rhythm, alternate the motion constantly from one hand to the other. Integrate these strokes with sweeping movements over the area.*

**5** *Return your hands to the lower back and place your thumbs each side of the spine, with your hands resting on the back at an angle to support the stroke. Slide your thumbs upwards firmly, applying enough pressure to ease tension out of the long muscles which support the spine. Finish by sweeping your hands out over the back of the neck and head.*

# Tender caresses...

WHEN THE BACK and shoulders feel thoroughly relaxed by deep and vigorous strokes, heighten the sensuality of the massage with this series of gentle sweeping movements that encompass the whole of the back.

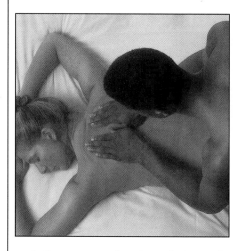

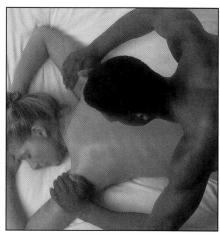

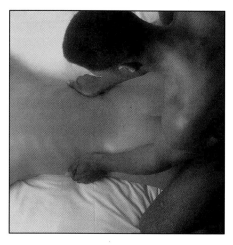

*1 Position your hands at the base of your partner's back on either side of the spine and slide them upwards. When your hands reach the upper back, mould them into your partner's shoulders as you draw them outwards.*

*Turn your wrists so your hands round smoothly over your partner's shoulders and upper arms. Then slide them back down the sides of her rib-cage and waist. As your hands pass over her skin, let them emphasize the shape of her body.*

*Move your hands back towards the source of your stroke, encircling the hips and buttocks as you do so. Repeat all these movements several times so they become one continuous fluid stroke around the back of her body.*

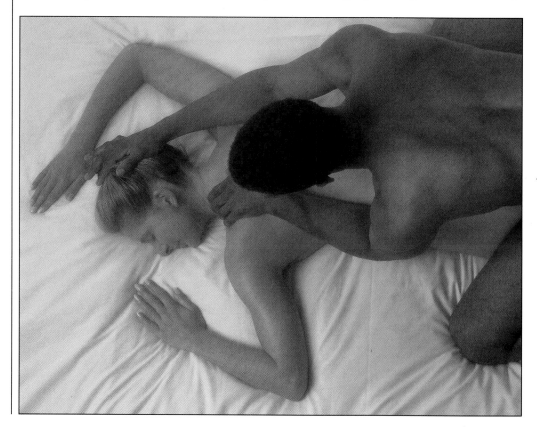

*2 Sweep your hands up the back and then continue to move one hand steadily up and over the neck and head as if you are brushing away the last residues of stress and tiredness. Tenderly rest your other hand on your partner's shoulder as you do this.*

**3** With your fingertips, massage over the back and sides of her head and scalp, using tiny but firm circular movements. This is a wonderful way to release tension from the scalp and to revitalize your partner. Ask her to turn her head and repeat these strokes on the other side, then stroke tenderly through her hair in a soothing and gentle way.

# Heightening the response . . .

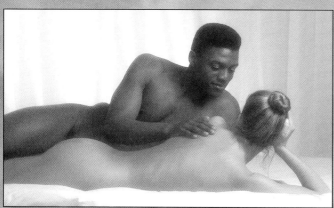

*Before you go on to massage your partner's front, let her enjoy the sense of release after your massage while you relax alongside her. If she wants to rest awhile, give her time to do so.*

ONCE YOU ARE BOTH ready to continue the massage, ask your partner to turn over so you can spread oil down her legs with soft, flowing strokes. Gently lift and open your partner's legs a little so they rest comfortably and feel relaxed at the joints. Massaging one leg at a time, use the long, upward sweeping strokes to cover the leg, hip and inner thigh before gliding your hands back down to the foot. During the following movements, coax your partner to relax completely and let you take charge. These leg stretches will give her a tremendous feeling of release.

1 *Start by taking your partner's left leg and placing your left hand firmly under her heel. Support her knee with your right hand. Push the leg slowly and steadily upwards from the heel and lift it from under the knee. When the knee is fully bent, slide your right hand over the top of it and gently push the leg towards your partner's body. This will create a deep stretch through the lower back, buttock and thigh.*

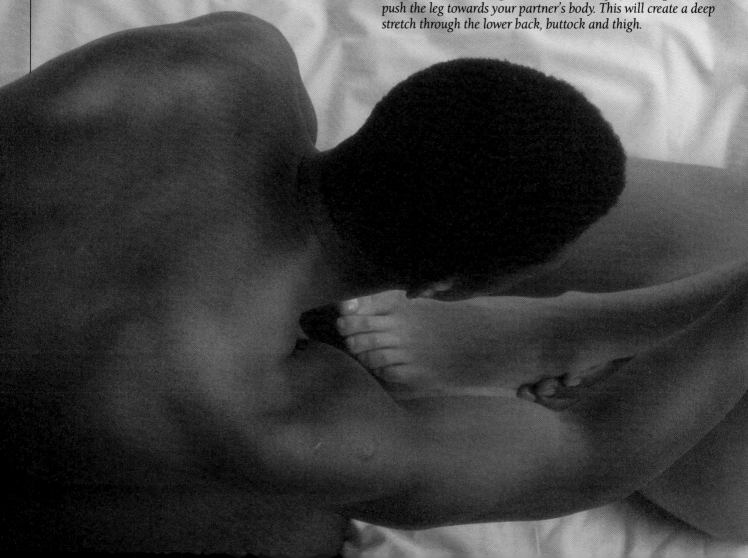

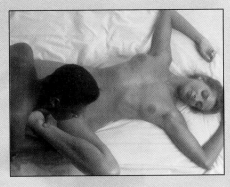

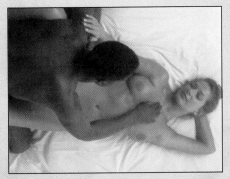

**2** Slide your right hand onto the outer thigh to support its weight. Slowly open the leg outwards, letting its weight fall into your hand. As your partner relaxes, tension will be released from her groin and inner thigh muscles. Slowly bring the leg back to a central position and return it to rest. Repeat all these movements on your partner's other leg.

**3** Move up closer to your partner's body, kneeling between her legs. Lean forwards to run your fingers over her chest and belly and down onto her thighs. Refreshed and revitalized, your partner will relish this playful stroking over her body.

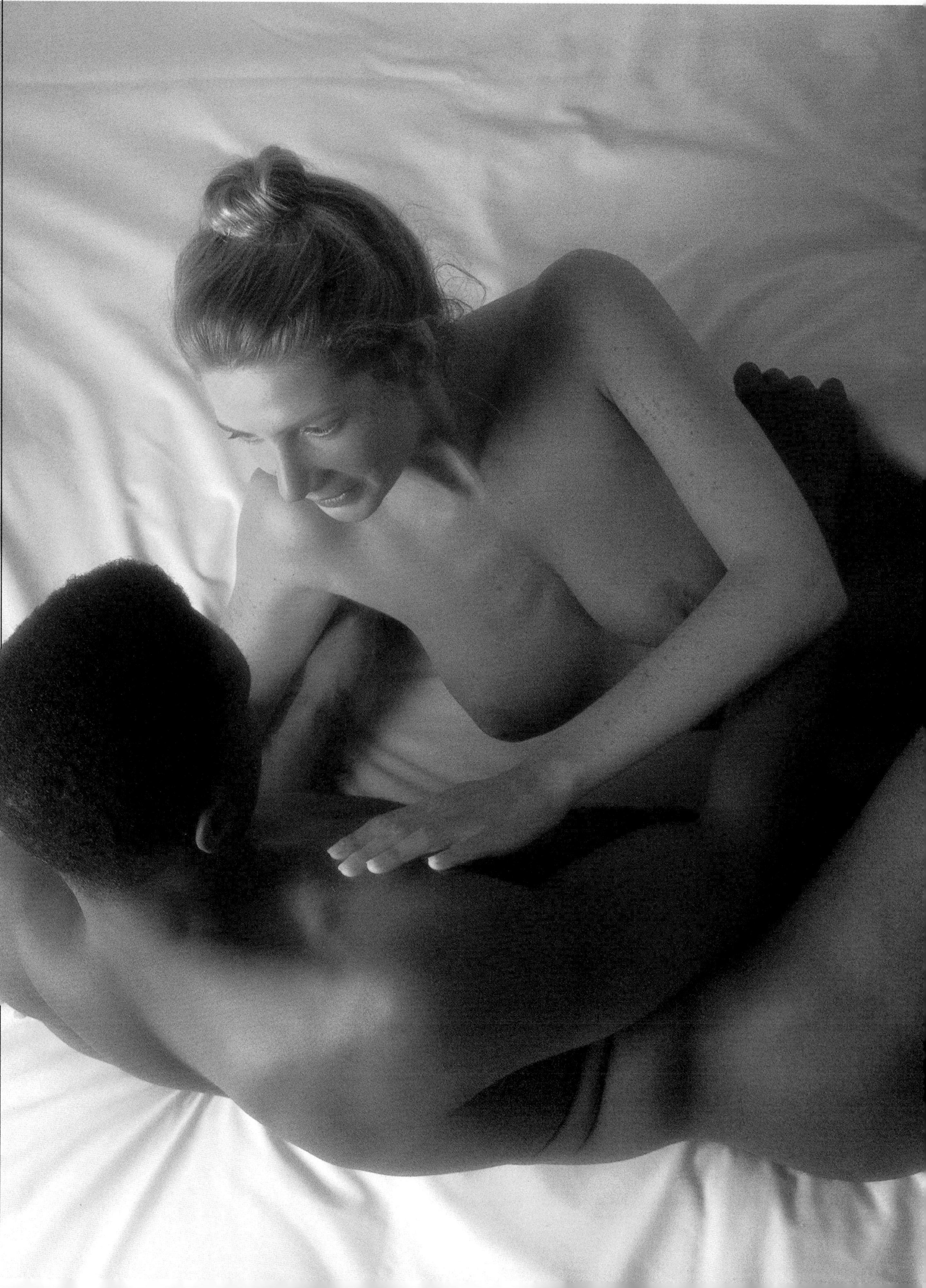

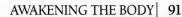

*When you are relaxed and in
harmony, you can find endless delight
and pleasure in each other . . .*

# Restorative massage

A QUICK MASSAGE over some of the most common tension areas – the back, shoulders, neck and head – can soothe away aches and tensions, revive flagging spirits, and enhance the feelings between you. There is no need for your partner to undress completely when having this massage, nor do you have to apply oil to your hands, which helps the informality and spontaneity of this sequence of strokes – you can do it anywhere at any time.

Have your partner sit or kneel in front of you. Alternatively, she can sit astride a chair, facing and using its back for support. Open the massage by simply placing your hands over your partner's shoulders. The warmth and comfort of your touch should help to melt away tensions so that the muscles start to relax.

**STARTING THE MASSAGE**

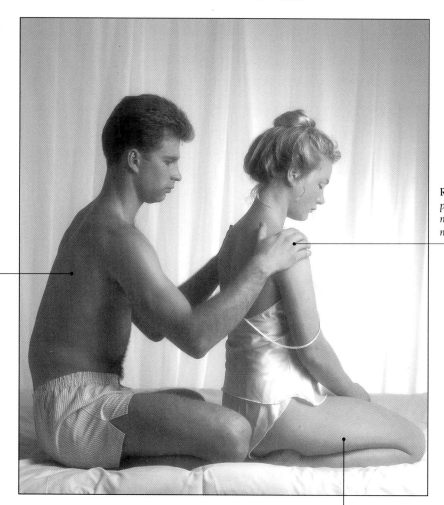

**Position yourself** *behind your partner so you can easily run your hands over her back and shoulders.*

**Rest your hands** *on your partner's shoulders for some moments before you start to massage.*

**Your partner** *should sit or kneel in front of you in a comfortable position.*

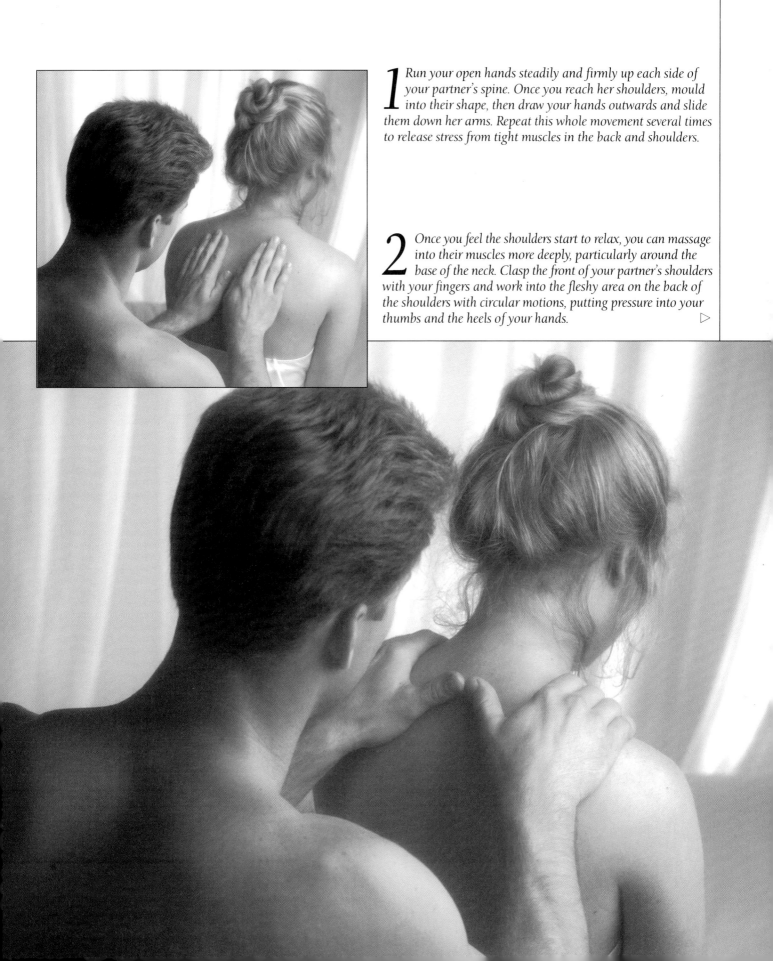

**1** Run your open hands steadily and firmly up each side of your partner's spine. Once you reach her shoulders, mould into their shape, then draw your hands outwards and slide them down her arms. Repeat this whole movement several times to release stress from tight muscles in the back and shoulders.

**2** Once you feel the shoulders start to relax, you can massage into their muscles more deeply, particularly around the base of the neck. Clasp the front of your partner's shoulders with your fingers and work into the fleshy area on the back of the shoulders with circular motions, putting pressure into your thumbs and the heels of your hands. ▷

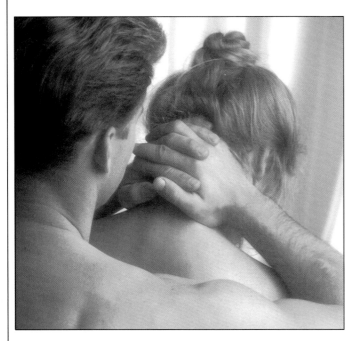

**3** Ask your partner to lean her head forwards so you can massage well into her neck muscles. With your fingers locked together, place your hands around the back of her neck, then draw the heels together slowly to squeeze the neck muscles gently, taking care not to drag the skin. Repeat this movement from the base to the top of the neck several times to help free tension and tightness.

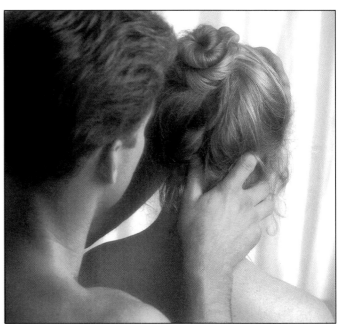

**4** Find the small hollow space that lies at the top of the spine, just below the skull. By pressing on this spot gently and steadily, you can help to alleviate headaches and stress. Support your partner's forehead with your left hand as you do this and place your right thumb pad into the hollow spot. Press in slowly and steadily with a slight upward movement for a few moments before releasing the pressure. Be sensitive as this can be a sore point.

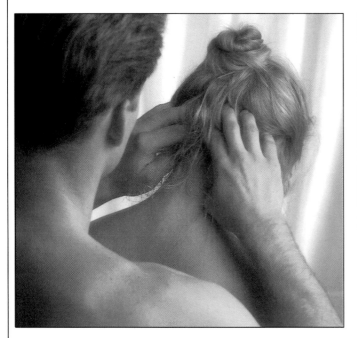

**5** Loosen and invigorate the scalp with tiny fingertip rotations, moving both hands over the back of the head from the base of the skull to the crown. This will refresh and revitalize your partner.

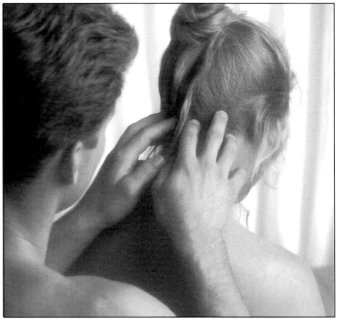

**6** Brush away any remaining stress by stroking your hands lovingly down your partner's head, the back of her neck and out over her shoulders several times. Continue to stroke down and out over her back.

**7** Now let your partner fall back into the support of your body. This simple act of letting go can help a deeper relaxation to take place. Stay together in this position for some moments.

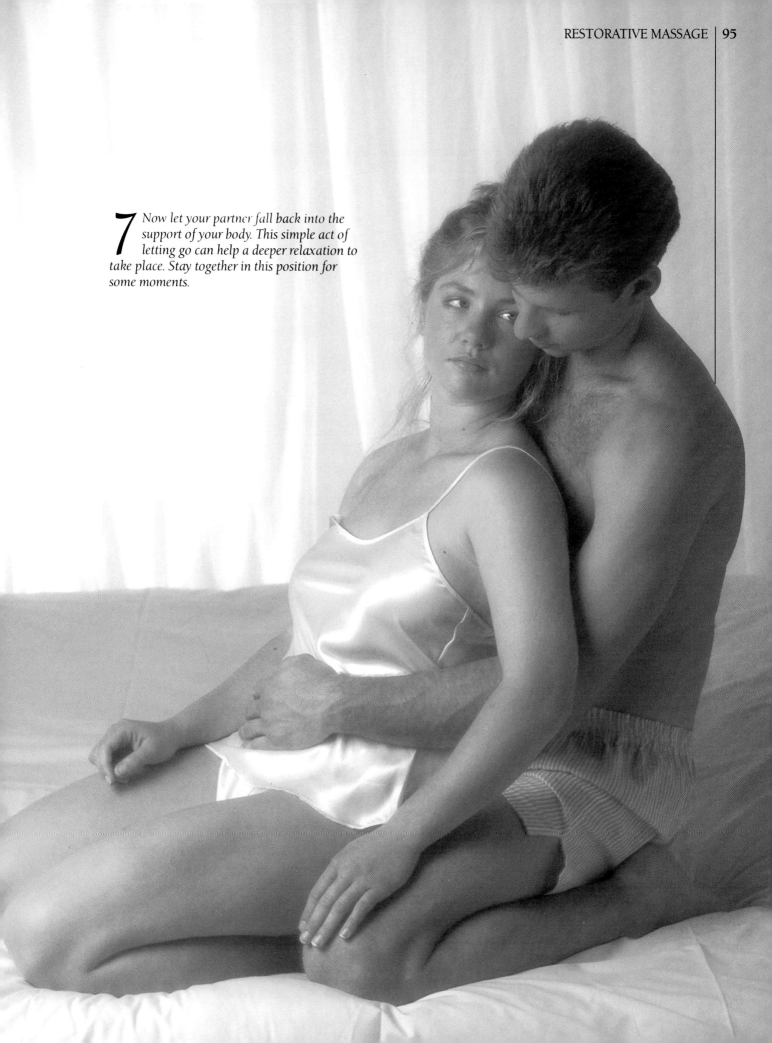

# Harmonizing holds

B Y SIMPLY TOUCHING and holding your partner's body at various points, you can impart a profound sense of wholeness, integration and balance. Such holds can introduce moments of stillness and calm into a massage, and provide you with the opportunity to rest as you move from one area of the body to another. They are also an effective way of comforting and relaxing your partner if he is anxious or sick, or at times when a full massage would be inappropriate.

As you lay your hands over different parts of your partner's body, close your eyes and become aware of your own breathing to increase the sensitive atmosphere of silence and stillness. If there are areas of pain or tension in his body, put your hands tenderly over them and imagine that through your touch alone, you are creating a healing, soothing and relaxing effect. Stay with each hold for as long as it feels appropriate to you, and always let your hands approach and leave the body gently. Follow a soothing pattern of holds moving from the head to the feet. A selection is shown here, but others feel equally good, such as hands over the top and bottom of the spine, or hands over the heart and the belly. Try other holds as your intuition directs.

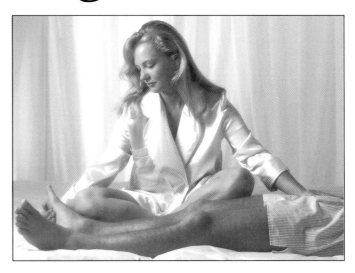

## THE BODY HOLD
*For a loving, intimate position that brings comfort and calm, ask your partner to curl up on his side in a foetal position. Snuggle up behind him and mould your own body into his shape. Place one hand on his belly and the other over the crown of his head, then rest together.*

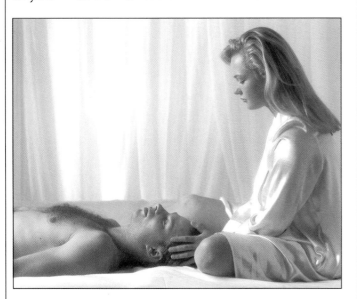

## THE CROWN
*Place your hands around the crown of your partner's head, so that your thumbs rest over his forehead and your fingers surround his scalp. This hold will have a calming effect on your partner, easing away strain and anxiety.*

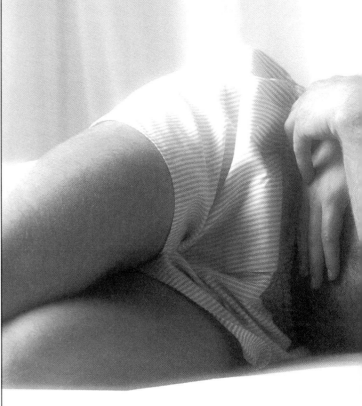

**THE HIP AND FOOT** *(opposite)*
*Sitting at your partner's side, place one hand on his hip and the other on the foot. This hold bestows a feeling of balance between the upper and lower parts of the body. You can produce a similar effect on the back of the body by holding the base of the spine and one foot.*

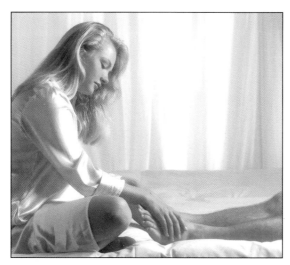

**THE FEET**
*Resting your hands over your partner's feet brings balance to his body and soothes away tension. This is an excellent way to complete a series of holds on both the front and back of the body.*

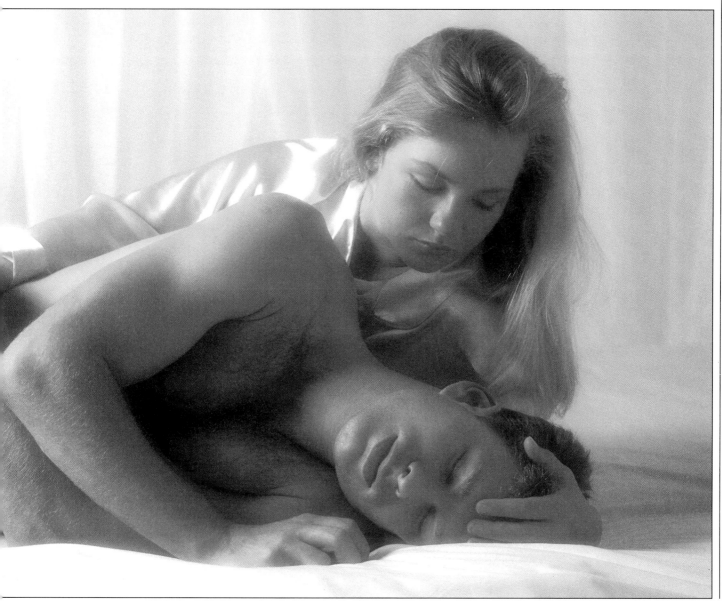

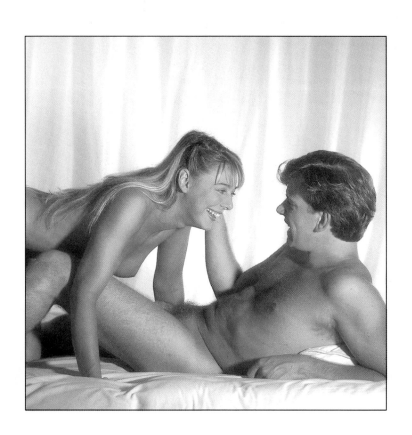

# The art
# of arousal

SEXUAL CONDITIONING tends to cast men as
active and women as passive, but there
should always be room for role reversal. In the
following programme, the man is receptive
while the woman delights in taking the
initiative to arouse him.
Male sexuality is often taken for granted when in
fact it is just as vulnerable as a woman's to
personal stress, tension and changes in health or
circumstances. Once a man feels free to relax
into receiving a sensual massage, not only is he
nourished by his partner's loving, tender touch, he
is also more able to tune into and accept his
more vulnerable and sensitive feelings. Conversely,
a woman can feel liberated and empowered by
taking the lead in a sexual relationship.
The following massage progresses up the body from
the feet to the belly, and is both relaxing
and stimulating. The sequence of strokes and playful
touches is equally enjoyable whichever partner
is giving or receiving the massage.

# Awakening sensuality...

THE FEET CONTAIN some surprisingly erogenous
zones, most particularly on the soft skin
between the toes and on the big toe itself. This massage
starts by relaxing the feet, one at a time, and
then moves on to more arousing strokes.
Start by spreading oil smoothly down each leg in
turn and over the feet, stroking down from
the hips and taking in the inner thighs too. If your
partner is very hairy, apply additional oil to
prevent pulling or tangling the hair when making
upward strokes. As a prelude to the massage,
rake your fingers down the legs and over
the feet several times.

## GETTING INTO POSITION

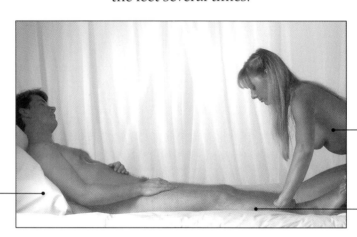

**Let your partner** *lie back, or be supported with cushions or pillows so that he can watch you massage.*

**Find a comfortable** *position to make your strokes. Change it whenever necessary.*

**Apply oil** *to each leg before you start to massage the foot.*

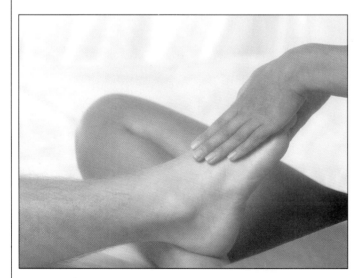

*1 Sitting at your partner's feet, rest the heel of one foot against your leg so you can touch the sole and the upper surface easily. Cradle and warm the foot between your hands for a few moments. Then, with both hands, stroke down the lower leg and over the foot. Repeat these soothing strokes to help your partner let go of any accumulated stress.*

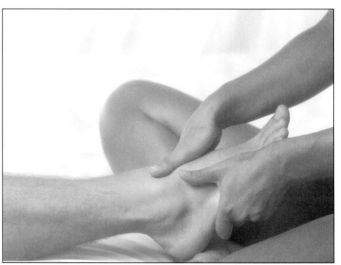

*2 Loosen the foot further by making circular strokes with your thumbs and the heels of your hands, one hand following the other. Place your fingers under the sole to support the movement and increase the pressure on the first half of each stroke. Massage from the base of the toes to the ankle, then slide your hand back and repeat several times.*

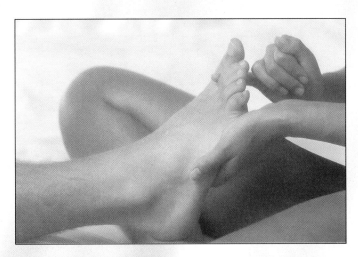

**3** *Run your little finger down the inside of each toe, lingering over the sensitive soft skin that lies in between, then stroke up the side of the next toe.*

**4** *Stimulate the big toe from its base to its tip by holding it between your thumb and forefinger, massaging upwards on the front and then the back by making small circles with your thumb. Concentrate on the pad of the big toe. Intensify any erotic sensations by varying the rhythm of your strokes.*

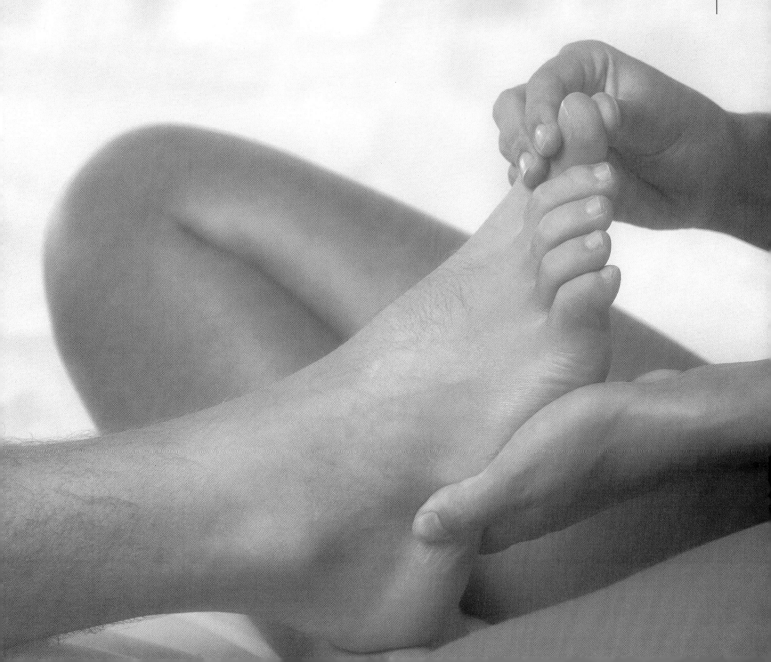

# Getting into a rhythm ...

AS YOU START TO SWEEP your hands up the legs, over the thighs and hips, mould your strokes into a continuous, fluid movement. Sway your body forwards into the upward strokes, and vary between softer and deeper pressure to intensify the pleasure and sensuality. Slow the pace to give your partner enough time to enjoy and experience the full sensations of your massage.

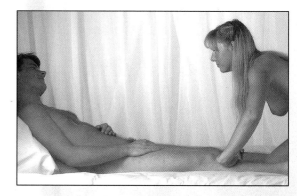

*1 Place one hand on the front of each foot, with your fingers facing inwards. Sweep both hands up the legs smoothly and firmly.*

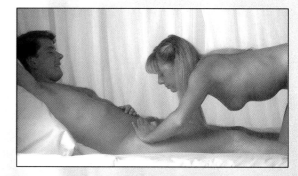

*2 Continue the stroke over the thighs and around the hips, then pull your body back and bring your hands down the back of the legs, sliding them under the heels and over the soles of the feet. Repeat this stroke over the legs several times, building up into a steady speed and rhythm.*

**3** Rest your hands just above your partner's knees so your fingers lie on the inner side of the legs. Stroke firmly up the insides of the thighs to the groin. Draw your fingers up over the loins until your hands encircle the pelvis, then slide your fingers just under the buttocks and glide them down under the thighs. Sweep your hands back over the knees so that your fingers return to the inside of the legs. Repeat in a continuous flowing motion.

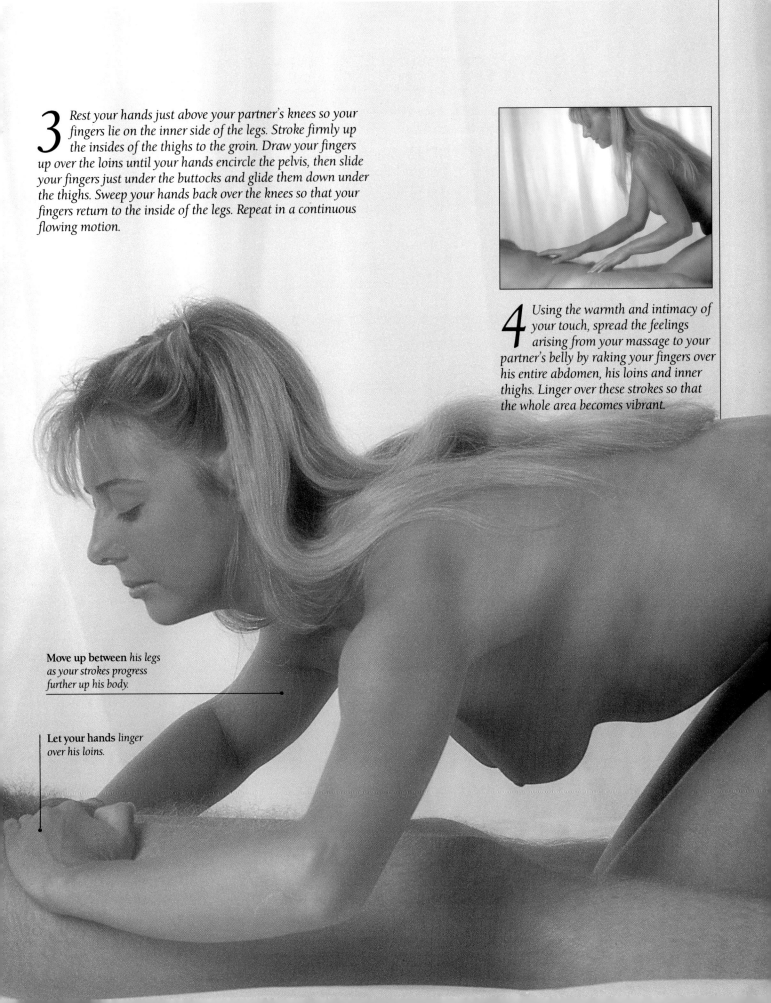

**4** Using the warmth and intimacy of your touch, spread the feelings arising from your massage to your partner's belly by raking your fingers over his entire abdomen, his loins and inner thighs. Linger over these strokes so that the whole area becomes vibrant.

**Move up between** *his legs as your strokes progress further up his body.*

**Let your hands** *linger over his loins.*

# Strokes for arousal ...

COVERING THE UPPER THIGHS with gentle but firm strokes invigorates and stimulates the whole of this area, often increasing arousal and sexual spontaneity.
Ask your partner to raise the knee of one leg so you can stroke all over and around his inner thigh. Ease any tension he may feel in his leg by placing a cushion under his hip or supporting his leg against your thigh. Massage one leg at a time, fusing the strokes shown below into the flow of your massage by sweeping your hands over the whole of the upper leg and hip area after each sequence.

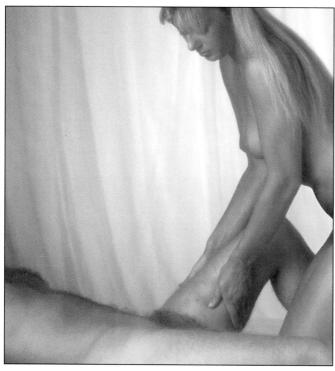

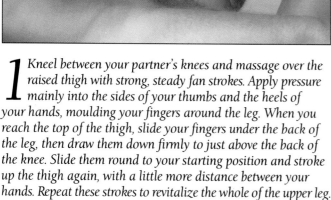

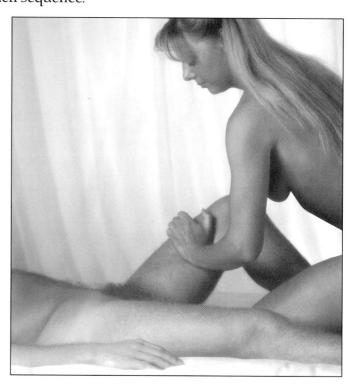

*1* *Kneel between your partner's knees and massage over the raised thigh with strong, steady fan strokes. Apply pressure mainly into the sides of your thumbs and the heels of your hands, moulding your fingers around the leg. When you reach the top of the thigh, slide your fingers under the back of the leg, then draw them down firmly to just above the back of the knee. Slide them round to your starting position and stroke up the thigh again, with a little more distance between your hands. Repeat these strokes to revitalize the whole of the upper leg.*

*2* *Support your partner's leg with one hand on the outer thigh as it opens and relaxes, exposing the inner thigh and groin for deeper massage. Place your other hand just above the knee and stretch along the inside thigh muscle in a steady movement towards the groin, applying pressure into the heel of your hand while keeping your fingers off the body. Sweep your full hand softly back down the inner thigh to where your stroke began. Repeat this stretch over the whole of the inner thigh to relax muscles which often hold sexual tension.*

*3* *As you feel the area mellow under your touch, make gentle but firm circles with your fingertips, moving into and along the groin.*

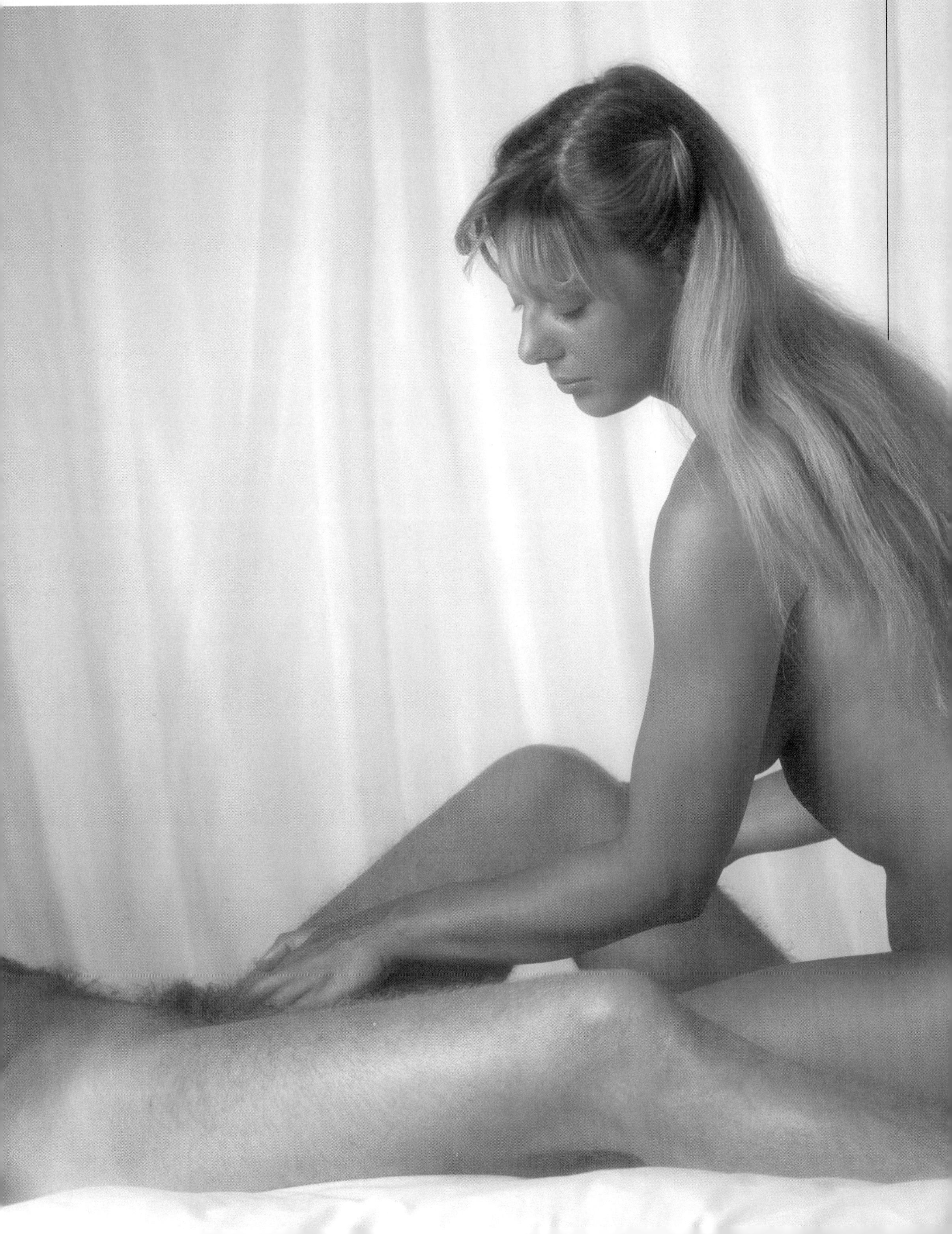

# Exciting play...

B Y NOW, the whole erogenous area surrounding
your partner's genitals should be relaxed yet
vibrant. As you kneel between his raised knees, his
position is both open and receptive.
Potentially, these are highly erotic
moments for you both.
Savour them, heightening the sensuality through
your touch and a deepening awareness
of each other.

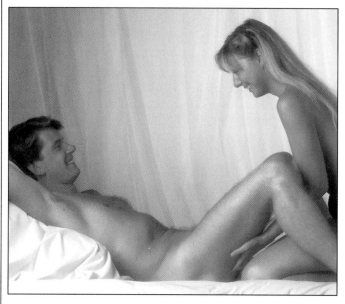

1 *Slip your hands a little under the buttocks and draw
your fingertips slowly down the underside of his thighs
several times. Linger over the soft skin, deepening the
pressure in the tips of your fingers as you slowly rake them
downwards. Tantalize this area further by stroking down the
underside of your partner's thighs with your fingernails. Then
ease the position of his knees so that his legs lie open,
fully relaxed.*

2 *Now cover the thighs and loins with feather-light finger
strokes, so light that at times you are barely touching his
skin. If your hair is long enough, excite him further by
sweeping it softly over his belly, thighs and genitals.*

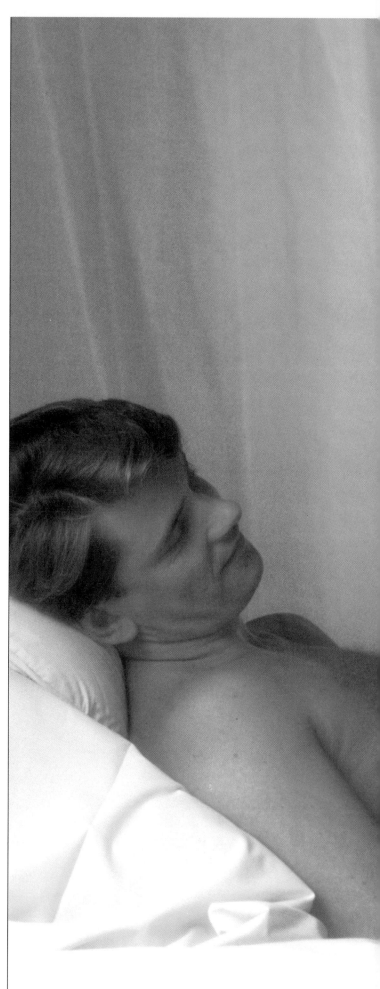

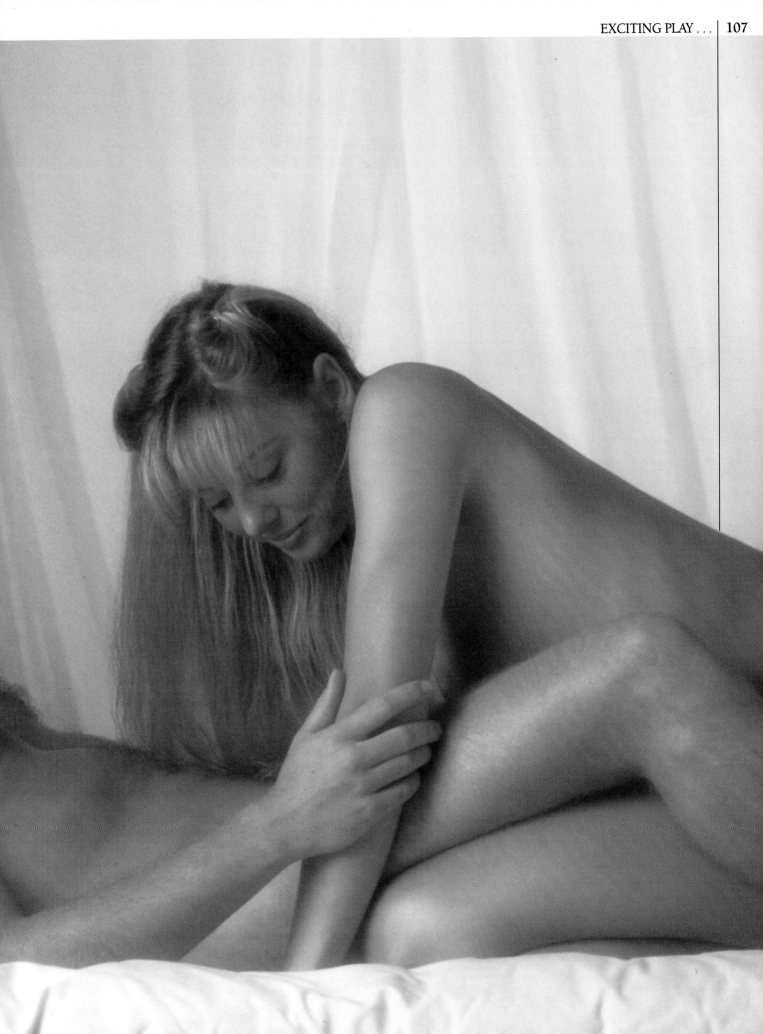

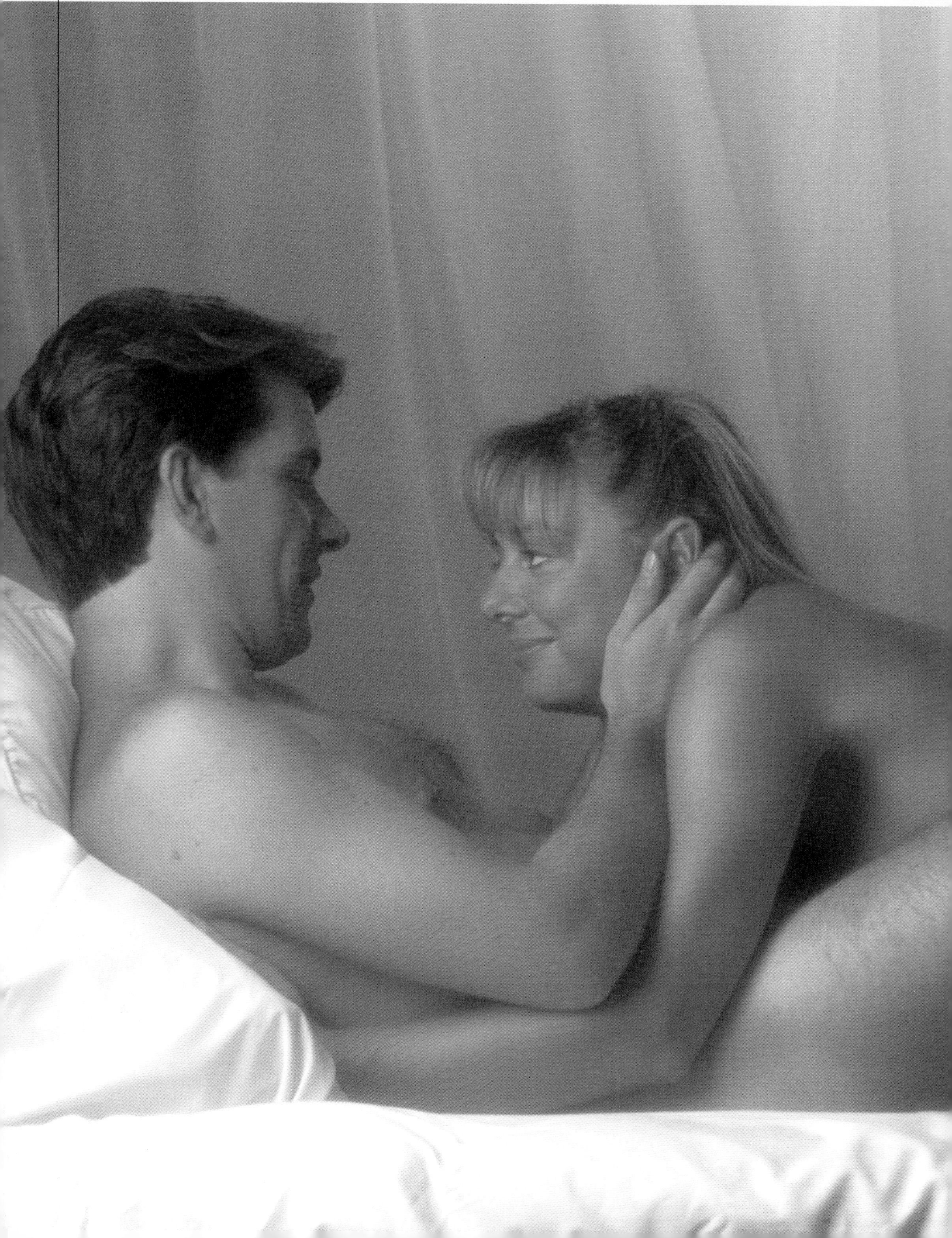

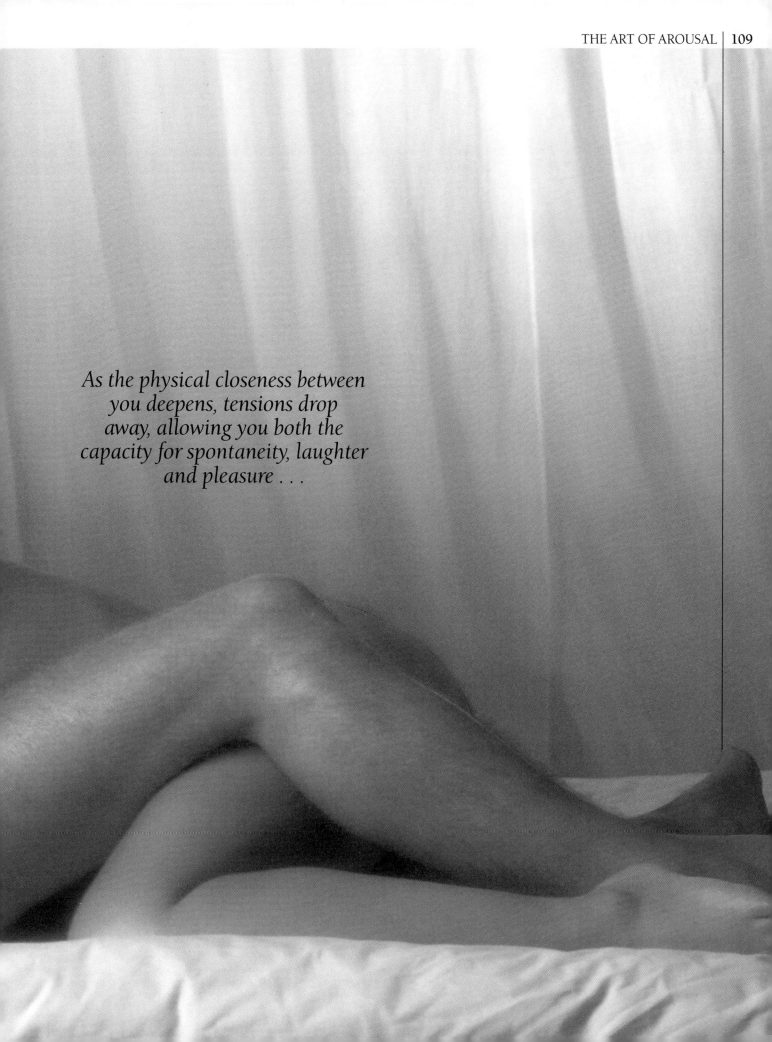

*As the physical closeness between you deepens, tensions drop away, allowing you both the capacity for spontaneity, laughter and pleasure . . .*

# Back massage

THE AREA SURROUNDING the spine frequently carries tension from day to day stress, emotional anxieties and incorrect posture. Yet a relaxed spine benefits the whole body, boosting energy and restoring a feeling of well-being. For times when your partner complains of a sore back, here is a sequence of effective strokes to ease away tension from these muscles. Repeat the movement shown in the first two steps several times until you feel the muscles softening under your hands, then go on to the deeper strokes.

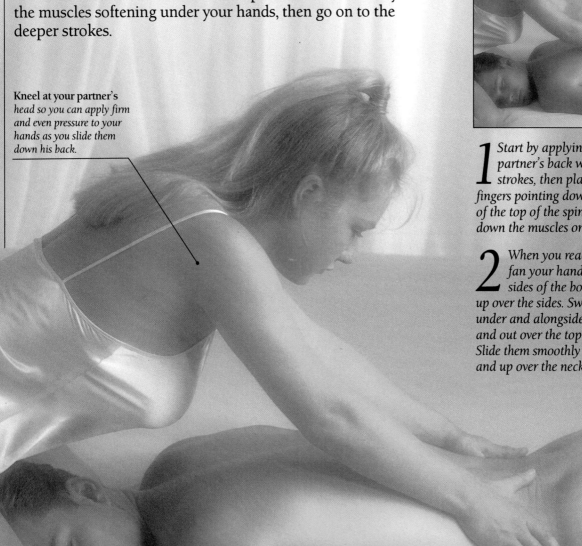

**Kneel at your partner's** *head so you can apply firm and even pressure to your hands as you slide them down his back.*

1 *Start by applying a little oil to your partner's back with soft, flowing strokes, then place your open hands, fingers pointing downwards, on each side of the top of the spine. Slide them firmly down the muscles on either side.*

2 *When you reach the lower back, fan your hands outwards to the sides of the body. Glide them back up over the sides. Swing them inwards, under and alongside the shoulder blades and out over the top of the shoulders. Slide them smoothly around the shoulders and up over the neck and head.*

**Fan your hands** *out to the sides of the body as they reach the lower back.*

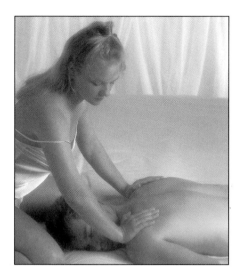

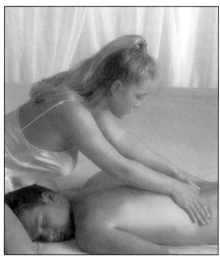

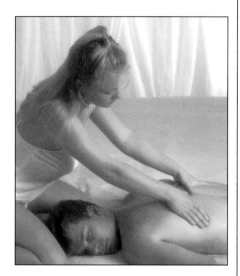

**3** *Release tension from your partner's shoulders by applying firm pressure. Place one hand over each shoulder and push down and outwards on each one alternately. Build up into a steady rocking motion as you repeatedly press on one shoulder then the other.*

**4** *Press your thumbs firmly into the grooves that lie on either side of the spine. Slide them downwards steadily, keeping the rest of your hands on the back. Return your hands to the top of the spine by sweeping them over and around the sides of the body and the shoulders. Repeat several times, increasing the pressure with each down stroke.*

**5** *Massage even deeper into the muscles alongside the spine by sliding your thumbs down one after the other, making short firm strokes. Work down one side of the spine then repeat the strokes down the other. If you feel a tense, tight spot, stroke your thumbs over it for some moments until you feel the area soften.*

**6** *A firm stretch motion down either side of the spine will relax your partner further. Place the heel of one hand at the top of the back on one side of the spine, keeping your hand and fingers straight and raised slightly off the body. Add weight to your stroke with your other hand. Slide downwards steadily as far as you can reach. Repeat this stroke down the muscles on the other side of the spine. Finish the massage by covering your partner's back with soothing, downward fan strokes.*

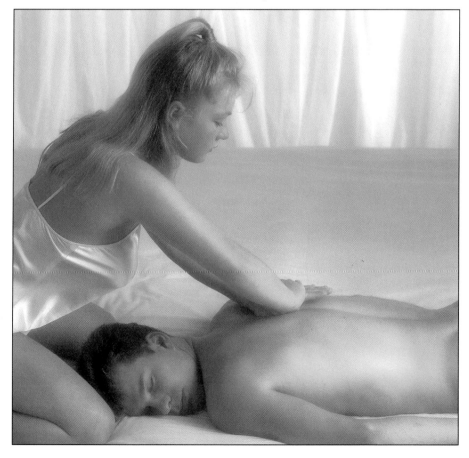

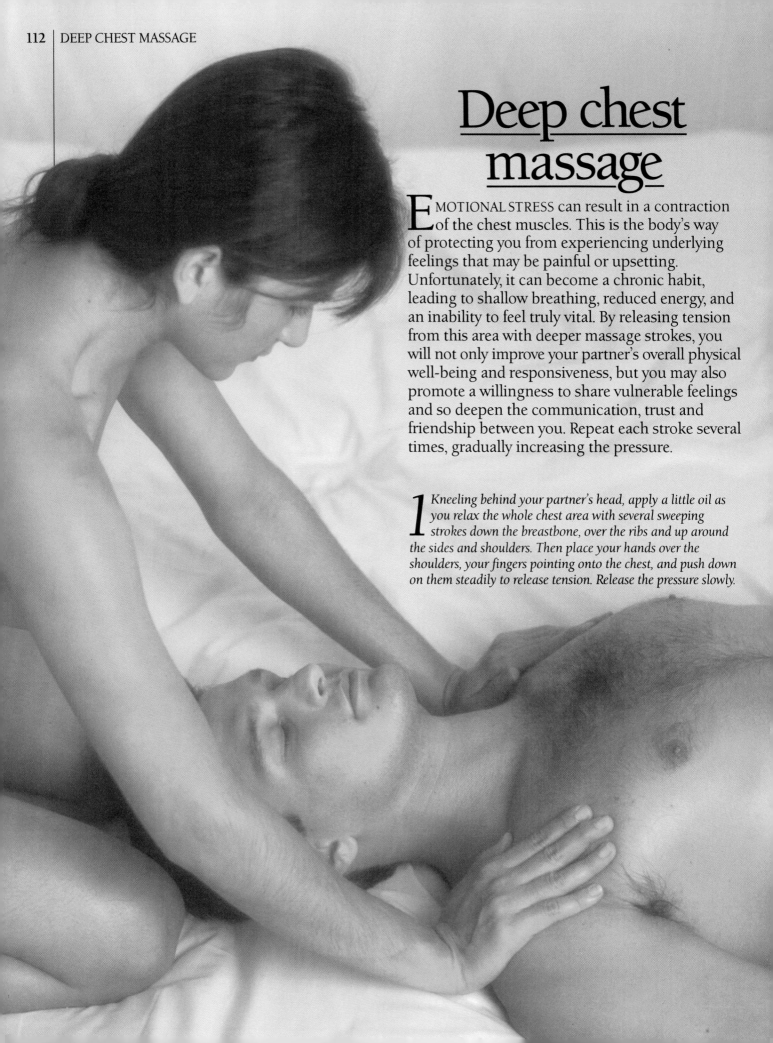

# Deep chest massage

EMOTIONAL STRESS can result in a contraction of the chest muscles. This is the body's way of protecting you from experiencing underlying feelings that may be painful or upsetting. Unfortunately, it can become a chronic habit, leading to shallow breathing, reduced energy, and an inability to feel truly vital. By releasing tension from this area with deeper massage strokes, you will not only improve your partner's overall physical well-being and responsiveness, but you may also promote a willingness to share vulnerable feelings and so deepen the communication, trust and friendship between you. Repeat each stroke several times, gradually increasing the pressure.

1 *Kneeling behind your partner's head, apply a little oil as you relax the whole chest area with several sweeping strokes down the breastbone, over the ribs and up around the sides and shoulders. Then place your hands over the shoulders, your fingers pointing onto the chest, and push down on them steadily to release tension. Release the pressure slowly.*

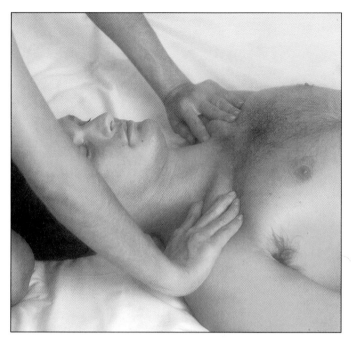

2 Relax the collar-bone by placing the tips of the first two fingers of each hand above and below the bone, firmly drawing them out towards the shoulders. Never put pressure on the bone itself.

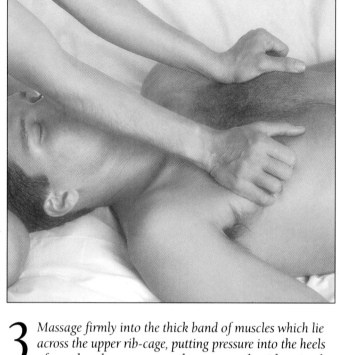

3 Massage firmly into the thick band of muscles which lie across the upper rib-cage, putting pressure into the heels of your hands as you move them outwards with a circular motion. Continue around the sides of the armpits.

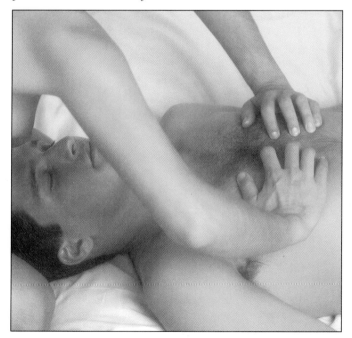

4 Loosen the tissue between the ribs by stroking your fingertips outwards from the breastbone to the sides. Bend your fingers to increase the pressure. These strokes will give your partner a feeling of expansion and release throughout his chest and rib-cage.

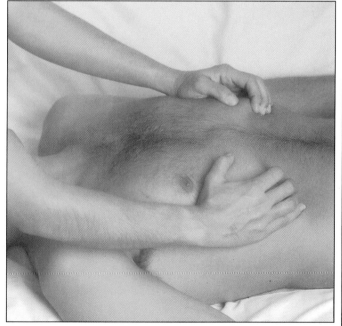

5 Tense muscles under the rib-cage can restrict full breathing. Once this area has begun to relax under softer massage strokes, sink your fingertips under the breastbone and then draw them gently but firmly outwards, stretching under the lower ribs towards the sides. Ease the pressure as you reach the sensitive areas at the sides of the rib-cage.

# Hand massage

HANDS ARE CAPABLE of great sensitivity, but they are usually so busy doing that they seldom relax into receiving. Consequently, a hand massage is always a sensual and comforting experience. It is a simple massage to give, requiring little time and preparation, and it can take place anywhere. Massage one hand at a time and support it with one of your own hands, transferring it to your other hand whenever necessary to make your strokes. Pamper dry and work-worn hands by massaging in a small amount of lotion as you make the following strokes.

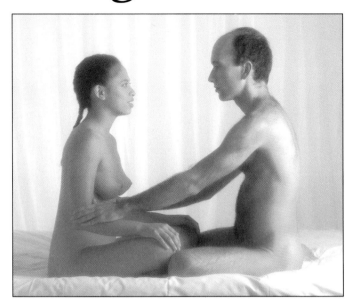

*1 Sit facing each other and open the massage by relaxing your partner, stroking your hands softly down from her neck, over her shoulders, down her arms and out over her hands. Repeat this stroke several times.*

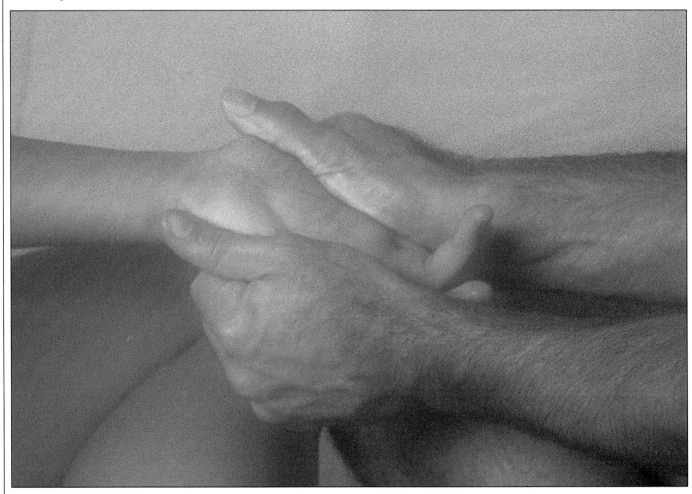

*2 Support one hand with the fingers of both your own hands placed beneath its palm. Begin by loosening the whole hand with a stretching movement. Draw your thumbs and heels firmly over the back of the hand, from the centre to the outer edges. Work up from the knuckles to the wrist and back down again several times. Turn the hand over and repeat these stretch strokes across your partner's palm, working from the base of the fingers to the wrist, and back.*

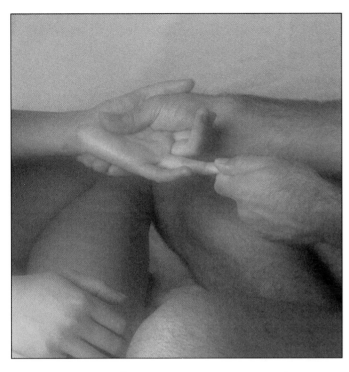

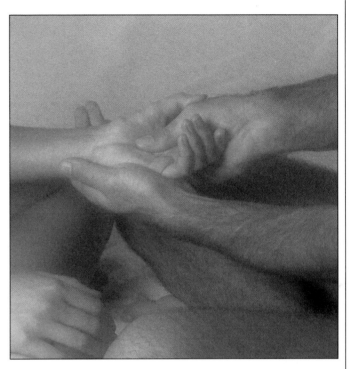

**3** *Grip the little finger at its base between your thumb and forefinger and pull firmly but gently along it several times, giving it an extra squeeze at its tip. Repeat on each finger, then change hands to pull along the thumb.*

**4** *Massage thoroughly and consistently over the base of the thumb and the surface of the palm, making circular motions with the tip of your thumb. Apply some pressure as you make these movements to penetrate the muscles.*

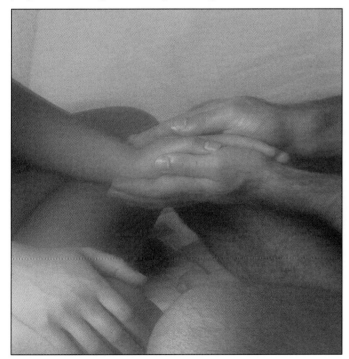

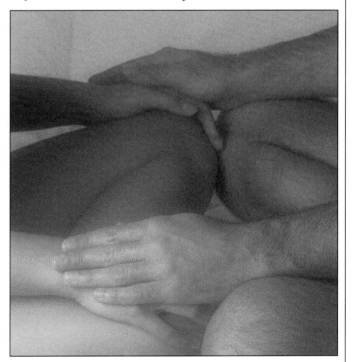

**5** *Place your partner's hand, with its palm facing downwards, between both your own hands and let it rest there for several moments in a warm, reassuring hold.*

**6** *Repeat all these strokes on your partner's other hand. Then glide your own hands down your partner's arms once more and bring them to rest over her hands. This is a soothing and loving way to finish your massage.*

# Special effects

IMAGINE THE COOL, delicate touch of pure silk on your skin, or the tantalizing brush of feathers against your body. For a playful and totally sensual experience, you and your partner can experiment with using soft, exotic materials in your massage to soothe, tease and heighten your responses to the barest of touches.

The most sensitive parts of the body to these light, erotic sensations are the areas of soft skin that are rarely exposed or touched. Trail luxuriant silk or velvet over the sides of the body, under the arms, along the inner thighs and the back of the knees. Or tantalize with gloriously coloured peacock feathers, or fluffy ostrich plumes, gently sweeping them over your partner's body from top to bottom, or vice versa. Vary the speed of these feather strokes from fast to very slow. Stroke behind the neck and softly over the face. Brush around the buttocks and linger over the thighs.

Perhaps your partner prefers a firm touch. While nothing can replace the benefits of a hands-on massage, you may like to experiment with the various massage implements now available. Wooden rollers, brushes and massage vibrators can all make interesting additions or alternatives to a regular massage and they have proved to be effective tools for stimulating or relaxing tense body muscles, or boosting the blood circulation.

For a totally uninhibited occasion, you and your partner could indulge in an exotic fruit massage. If you need an excuse, you can say you are using the fruit for its skin-healing properties (but do check first for allergies). Bathe and prepare your bodies for the event. Use sheets which are clean but replaceable. Squeeze the pulp of strawberries or apricots, or sweet-scented tropical fruits such as ripe mangoes or papayas, between your hands and treat it as a lotion, smoothing it all over each other's body. When you are ready to clean it off, take a shower together . . . or have a feast.

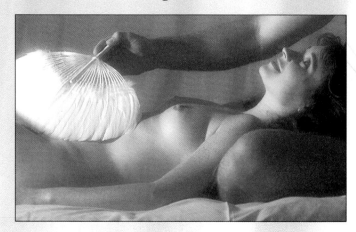

**Feather fan strokes**
*Be teased and tickled by the gentle brushes of a feather fan against your skin. Such soft strokes feel delicious, making the whole body alive and responsive.*

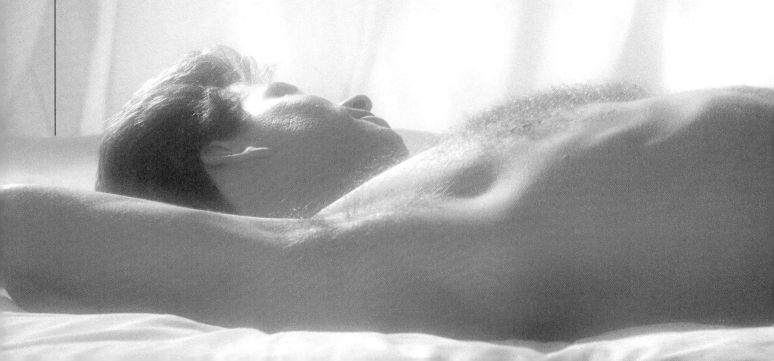

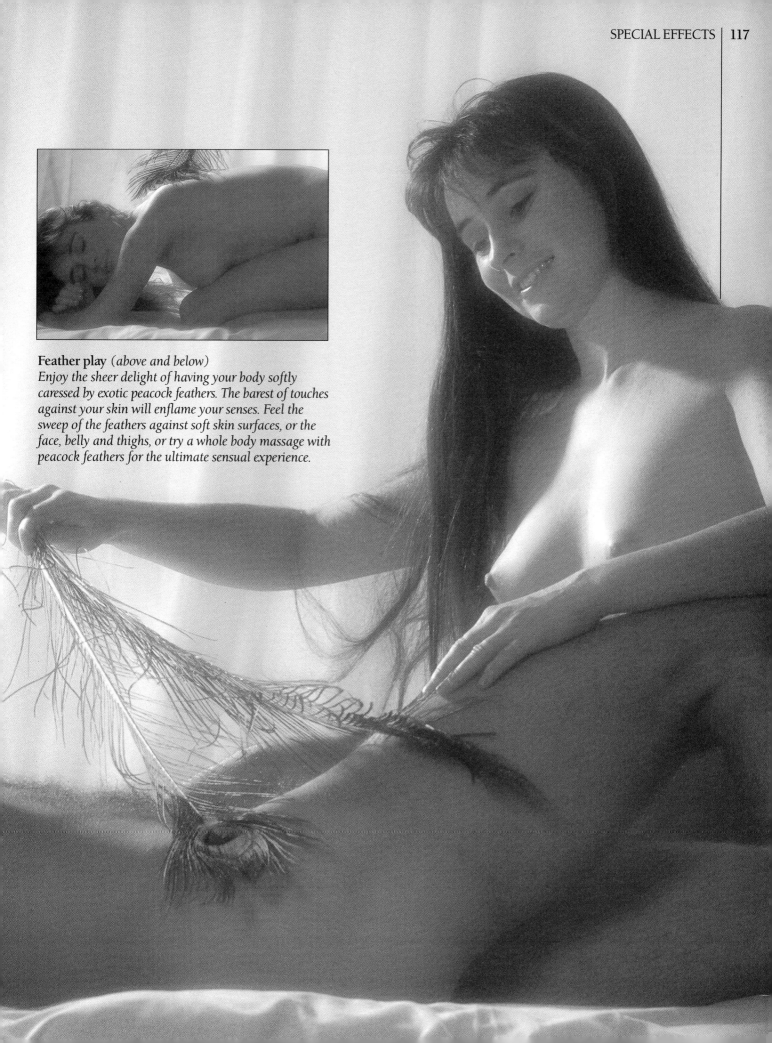

**Feather play** *(above and below)*
*Enjoy the sheer delight of having your body softly caressed by exotic peacock feathers. The barest of touches against your skin will enflame your senses. Feel the sweep of the feathers against soft skin surfaces, or the face, belly and thighs, or try a whole body massage with peacock feathers for the ultimate sensual experience.*

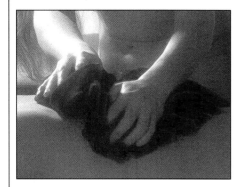

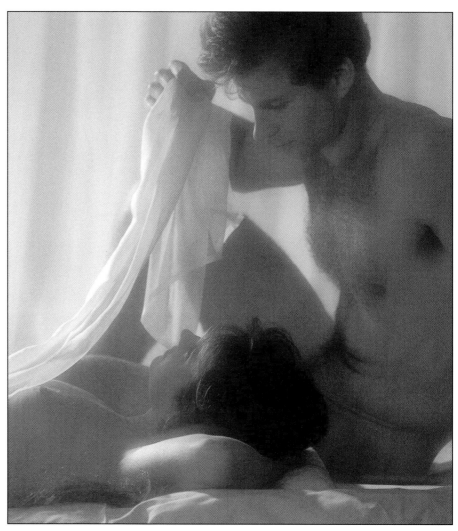

## Velvet

*Experiment and develop the sense of touch by seeing how your partner responds to the feel of different textures. Rub or brush velvet all over the body to experience its rich, soft fabric. Play with other materials and enjoy the varying sensations they bring as you trail and stroke them over each other's body.*

## Silk

*The soft, natural luxuriance of silk imparts its cool, smooth texture to the body, when gently trailed across sensitive areas of skin. The delicate touch of silk feels wonderful against the neck and belly, under the arms and over the thighs.*

**Chiffon** *(above and opposite)*
*Chiffon is delicate, translucent and light as air. It feels exciting when drawn gently over the skin. Play with it, letting it touch, caress and brush the breasts, the thighs and the sides of the neck. Rub it softly back and forth against the body.*

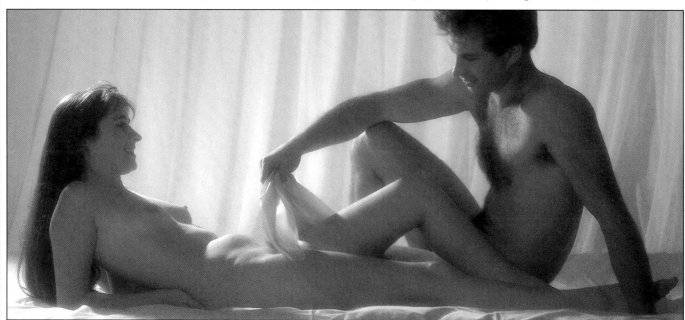

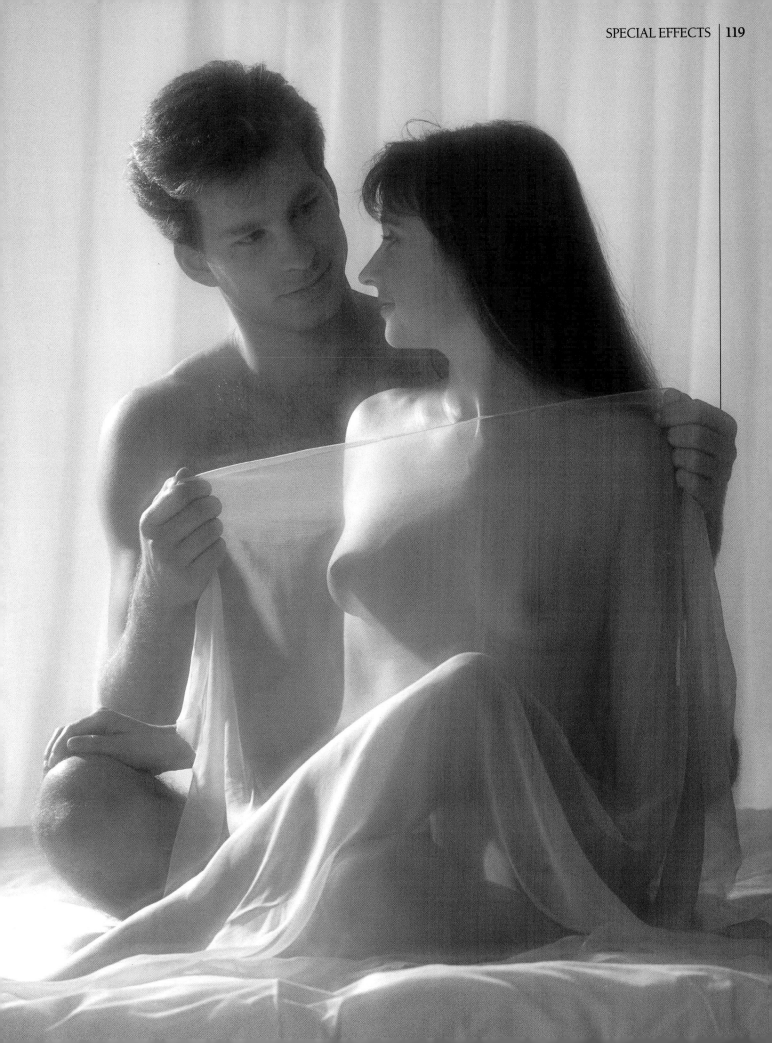

# Mutual massage

**M**AKE THE MOST of any opportunity to turn a tender touch or caress into a sensual mutual massage. Such moments can produce an overwhelming feeling of togetherness.

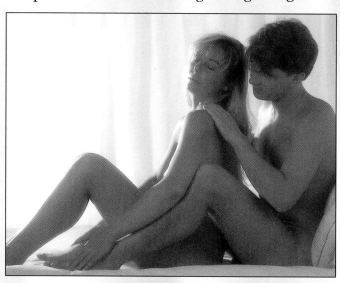

*1 In this comfortable and intimate position, you can relax your partner's shoulders with a simple massage while she makes light, soothing strokes over your feet.*

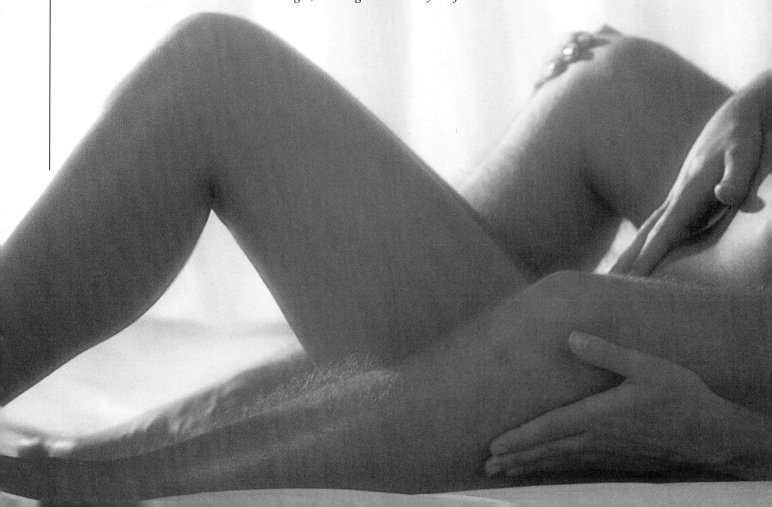

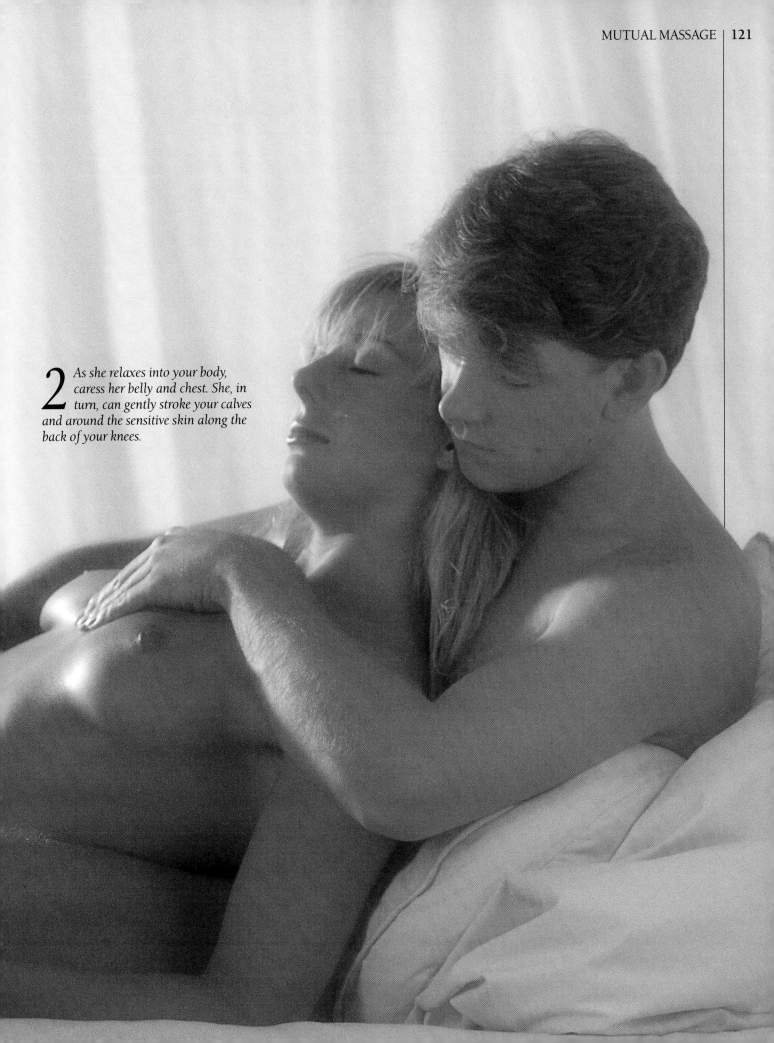

**2** As she relaxes into your body, caress her belly and chest. She, in turn, can gently stroke your calves and around the sensitive skin along the back of your knees.

# Mutual massage

LET YOUR TOUCHING be a journey of discovery over the hills, curves and valleys of your partner's body. Feel the texture of the skin, the bones and muscles, the heat changes and sensations created by your touch. Take time together and share your love. These moments of leisurely touching and stroking encourage feelings of closeness and serenity, deepening the intimacy between you.

*1 Lying side-by-side and face-to-face is a relaxing and intimate position in which to spend time together. You can gently touch and caress each other, moulding your hands over curves and tenderly tracing around features.*

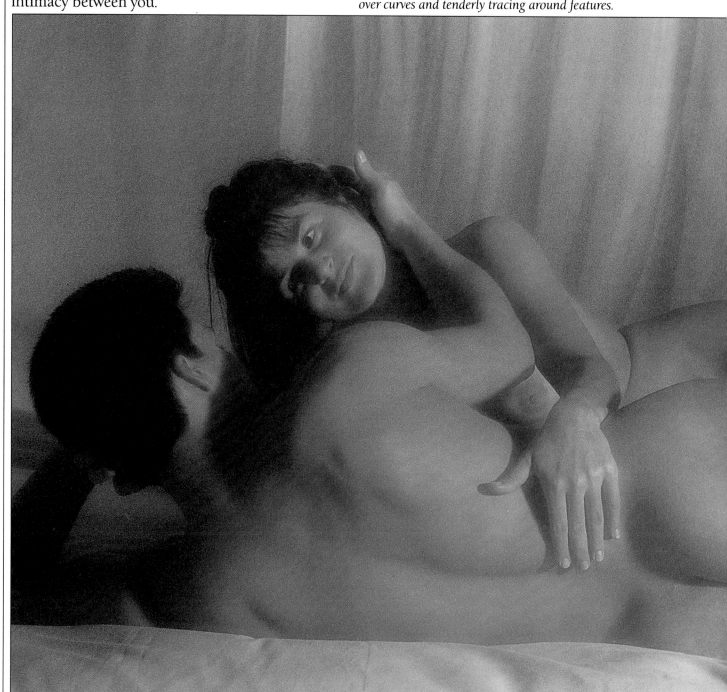

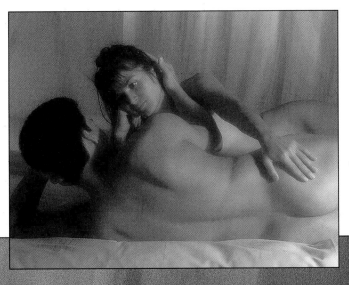

**2** *Such times of physical closeness, which allow for eye contact and gentle mutual caressing, will help you to open up to each other and develop a richer level of sharing between you.*

# Mutual massage

EVERY PART OF THE BODY is sensitive to touch, and those areas that do not receive much contact or attention, such as the back or the arms, can feel exquisitely responsive when caressed. While we are all familiar with communicating face-to-face, we seldom think to explore the possibilities of getting to know one another's bodies back-to-back. Try sitting together in the position shown here and simply familiarize yourselves with the feel of each other's back.

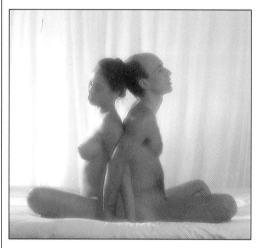

*1 Let your backs move gently together as if they are joined in a slow dance. Spend some time doing this. Feel the whole surface of your partner's back moving against your own. Become aware of all the sensations; of the skin, the pelvis, the spine, and the shoulders as they touch and rub softly against your own.*

*2 After gently moulding your backs together for several minutes, lean forwards so you can take your partner's weight and he can relax by stretching his body backwards over the surface of your own back.*

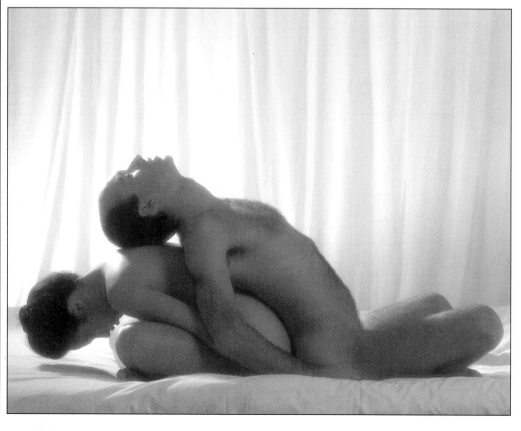

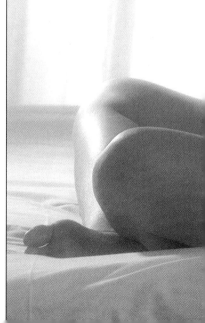

3 *Take it in turns to stretch your spines and release your shoulders fully. Hold the position only for as long as it is comfortable for you both.*

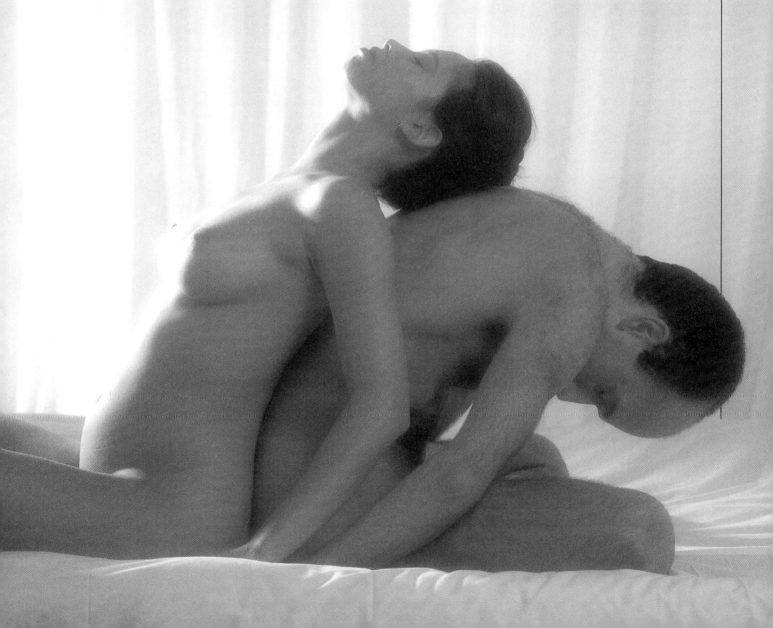

# Index

# Acknowledgments

**Author's acknowledgments**
I would like to thank Mano Collinge
for her inspiration and ideas,
and Linda Harness for the
aromatherapy recipes.

**Dorling Kindersley**
would like to extend their thanks
to all the models; Pamela Cowan,
who assisted Antonia Deutsch;
Gail Jones for helping with design;
Mike Hearn for retouching; and
Hilary Bird for the index.

**Photography**
All photography by Antonia Deutsch except:
pages 12-13  Dave King
Jacket flap  Tim Streater

**Make-up**
Bettina Graham

**Typesetting**
Modern Text, Southend-on-Sea
Set in Berkeleley Old Style

**Reproduction**
Colourscan, Singapore

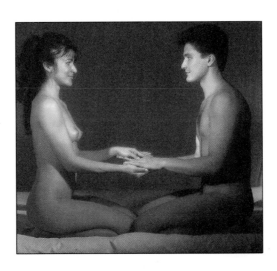